The Art of Cooking
for the Diabetic

The Art of Cooking for the Diabetic

Katharine Middleton
and
Mary Abbott Hess

Contemporary Books, Inc.
Chicago

Library of Congress Cataloging in Publication Data

Middleton, Katherine.
   The art of cooking for the diabetic.

   Includes index
   1. Cookery for diabetics.   I. Hess, Mary Abbott, joint author.   II. Title.
RC662.M53   1978   641.5′638   77-23701
ISBN 0-8092-8270-4 (cloth)
ISBN 0-8092-7222-9 (paper)

The use of brand names in this book is for product
identification only and does not constitute an endorsement by authors or publisher.

Published by Contemporary Books, Inc.
180 North Michigan Avenue, Chicago, Illinois 60601
Manufactured in the United States of America
Library of Congress Catalog Card Number: 77-23701
International Standard Book Number: 0-8092-8270-4 (cloth)
                                                  0-8092-7222-9 (paper)

Published simultaneously in Canada by
Beaverbooks
953 Dillingham Raod
Pickering, Ontario L1W 1Z7
Canada

Contents

Foreword

The Art of Cooking for the Diabetic provides a truly sound and exciting adventure for individuals who have diabetes, or for individuals who care for family members with diabetes. The knowledgeable authors, Katharine Middleton and Mary Abbott Hess, have carefully engineered this adventure by writing a book for diabetics that presents basic dietary principles and information, along with a volume of tasty recipes.

The book is beautifully structured. It begins with a glossary of terms used in diabetic dietetics and management to better inform and aid the reader. The diabetic diet is discussed in a comprehensive manner; this includes an extensive inventory of food exchanges to offer the diabetic a wide range in selection of foods, while maintaining his or her prescribed diet. The text contains an extraordinary section, "Living with Diabetes." Within it are discussed a number of items, unusual in a dietetic book, such as the influence of activity and sports upon diabetes, eating out (including exchanges for "fast food" operations), traveling, and sugar substitutes. Finally, the exceptional number of marvelous recipes with their food values per serving are detailed in the text. The recipes will win over the palates of a number of individuals without diabetes!

Kay Middleton and Mary Abbott Hess are professional nutritionists with outstanding credentials. They have given us a book that is complete in its dietary approach, most helpful in its discussion of "Living with Diabetes," and exceptional in its recipes.

The authorship of this fine text must be added to their long lists of honors.

Wesley H. Gregor, M.D.
Assistant Professor (Clinical) Medicine
Northwestern University Medical School
Formerly First Vice President, American Diabetes
  Association Northern Illinois Affiliate, Inc.

Acknowledgments

The authors are grateful for the sincere interest, practical suggestions, and generous assistance given to us by: the Home Economics Department of Mundelein College, Chicago; Mundelein students, especially Nancy Vesely; Eleanor Hess; Mark Thomas, Director of Marketing, and Reba Staggs, Director of Home Economics, National Live Stock and Meat Board; Bob E. Finley, Director of the Fisheries Education Center, National Marine Fisheries, U.S. Department of Commerce; Dorothy Holland, Vice President, Consumer Relations, Kraft, Inc.; Kathleen D. Preziosi, Sensory Education Specialist, Beatrice Foods Company; Ruth Musgrave, our patient and skillful typist; Janet Regan Klich, R.D., M.S. for providing ideas and nutrient data; Jeanette L. White, R.D., M.S. Nutritionist of the Northern Illinois Affiliate, American Diabetes Association, Inc., whose interest and comments were of special value; Mary's family (Peter, Rachel, Leslie, and Jo) and our friends who taste-tested loyally; and our diabetic friends, family, and patients who asked the questions that this book tries to answer. To one and all we hope this book will justify and fulfill your confidence in us.

Introduction

This book has been developed and written with loving care and much attention. The loving care included special attention to cooking techniques, the blending of food flavors, presenting food attractively, and above all, the art of cooking especially for the diabetic. The much attention has been in regard to giving the correct information on diabetes mellitus and its modern management, especially in regard to food selection. It is a response to the many questions we have been asked by diabetics and presents far more material and supplementary food lists than have ever been available before.

Both of us have years of experience as nutrition educators in classrooms, as speakers to women's groups, and at a professional level teaching nurses and students of dietetics. We have each counseled diabetics individually and in small groups. We have been active members of the Nutrition Committee of the Northern Illinois Affiliate, American Diabetes Association, Inc.

Mary has testified at several federal hearings in support of the expansion of diabetes education, diabetic counseling in patients' homes, and funding for diabetes research. Kay has been a very active volunteer and a member of the Board of Directors of the Northern Illinois Affiliate of the American Diabetes Association, Inc.

Our great interest in the whole area of diabetes and its management is very personal. Kay has been a diabetic for many years. Mary has several family members with diabetes.

Katharine Middleton

Mary Abbott Hess

1

Word Power

Alcohol: A substance produced when carbohydrates are fermented; provides 7 calories per gram; read Chapter 13, "Alcohol for Diabetics?"

Amino Acids: Proteins are made up of these.

Atherosclerosis: Deposits of fat and other substances in the walls of arteries which cause loss of elasticity and decreased blood flow.

Blood Sugar: The level of glucose in the blood which can be determined by a simple lab test.

Brittle: A term used to describe a form of diabetes that is particularly sensitive to changes in blood sugar and insulin levels; sometimes called **Labile, Unstable, Insulin Sensitive,** or **Juvenile Diabetes.**

Calorie: A unit to measure heat or energy provided by food; carbohydrate, proteins, fats, alcohol, and sugar alcohols provide calories; vitamins, minerals, and pure cellulose do not provide calories.

Carbohydrates: Compounds containing carbon, hydrogen, and oxygen found in sugars and starches; they yield 4 calories per gram and are a major source of energy for the body; read Chapter 19, "The Great Sugar Masquerade." The abbreviation for carbohydrate in our recipes is **CHO.**

Cardiovascular: Referring to the heart and blood vessels.

Cholesterol: A fatlike substance (sterol) found in animals; a part of the brain, hormones, cells, bile, nerve tissue, and blood; when too much is present it deposits in artery walls to cause atherosclerosis.

Diabetes Mellitus: The failure of body cells to use carbohydrates due to lack of insulin in a usable form; it is often referred to simply as diabetes.

Diabetologist: A doctor who specializes in the treatment of individuals with diabetes mellitus.

Diet Counselor: The dietitian, nutritionist, or physician who calculates, personalizes, and teaches the diabetic diet and other special diets.

Dietetic Foods: Foods for special diets, including low-sodium, fat-modified, water-packed, or sugar-reduced foods; not necessarily intended for diabetic diets; read Chapter 17, "How to Read a Label."

Enrichment: The addition of nutrients to a food to increase the consumption of those nutrients; enriched bread has added thiamin, riboflavin, niacin, and iron.

Fat: Oily substance found in meat, fish, poultry, eggs, cheese, milk, and some vegetables; a concentrated source of calories yielding 9 calories per gram; read Chapter 6, "Fat Exchanges" for a discussion of types of fat.

Fiber: Also called **Cellulose;** indigestible carbohydrates that are found in whole grains, nuts, fruits, and vegetables; after digestion they yield bulk but no calories.

Food Exchange: Lists of foods with similar nutrient values; read the section entitled "Exchange? What is That?" in the introduction to Part II, "The Diabetic Diet."

Food Habit: Your pattern of choosing and cooking the foods you have learned to eat; a result of cultural, economic, family, and religious influences.

Fortification: The addition of nutrients to foods that do not naturally have those nutrients; milk is often fortified with Vitamins A and D; many cereals, breakfast drinks, and man-made foods are fortified.

"Free": Containing few calories and carbohydrates; foods which may be used in the diabetic diet without controlling quantity, or which may be used in limited quantities without counting as an Exchange.

Gastrointestinal: Referring to the entire digestive tract.

Glucagon: A hormone produced by the pancreas that raises blood sugar by breaking down glycogen in the liver; its activity is opposite that of insulin.

Glucose: A simple sugar; read Chapter 19, "The Great Sugar Masquerade."

Glycemia: Sugar in the blood; if too high it is called **Hypergly-cemia;** if too low it is called **Hypoglycemia.**

Glycogen: Stored form of sugar in the liver.

Gram: A unit of weight in the metric system; one ounce is 28.35 grams on the scale. The abbreviation for gram is **gm.** in the recipes.

Hormone: A chemical produced by a gland or tissue and carried to other places in the body where it stimulates action.

Ideal Weight: The best weight of an individual based on sex, height, and bone structure; people of ideal weight statistically live longer and are healthier; also called **Desirable Weight.**

Insulin: A hormone produced by the beta cells of the pancreas; regulates the glucose going from the blood into body cells.

Juvenile Diabetes, or **Insulin-Requiring Diabetes:** Usually occurs early in childhood or adolescence; must be controlled by injections of insulin and diet; sometimes called **Brittle** or **Labile Diabetes.**

Low-Sodium Diet: Refers to a modified diet that may be prescribed by a physician. If your physician orders a specific amount of sodium, the diet counselor will help with your meal plans and may mark this book to help you select foods and recipes to give you the right amount of sodium. Follow the directions at the bottom of each recipe if you are on a low-sodium diet. This diet may also be called a **Salt-Free, Low-Salt,** or **Sodium-Restricted Diet.**

Low-Sodium Food: Foods that are processed or prepared without the addition of salt or other sodium products. Since most high-sodium foods contain salt (sodium chloride) such foods may also be labeled **Unsalted, Salt-Free,** or **Dietetic Low Sodium** when they are modified to be low in sodium. When foods are high in sodium (Worcestershire sauce, cereals, catsup, baking powder, cheese, etc.), a low-sodium product may be available in the diet food section of your grocery store.

Maturity Onset Diabetes: Diabetes that begins in adulthood; may be controlled by diet alone, oral hypoglycemic agents and diet, or insulin and diet; usually less severe than juvenile diabetes.

Meal Plan: A guide showing the number of Exchanges to use at each meal to properly distribute calories, carbohydrate, protein, and fat throughout the day; it is planned specifically for an individual by the diet counselor with consideration of dietary prescription and food habits of the individual.

Metabolism: The chemical and physical processes of all cells of the body.

Milligram: A metric weight equal to 1/1000 of a gram Sodium is measured in milligrams, the abbreviation for which is **mg.**

Mineral: Chemically inorganic substances found in nature that are needed in small amounts to build and repair body tissue or control metabolism.

Monounsaturated Fat: Contains primarily neutral fat which doesn't influence blood cholesterol; olive and peanut oils are primarily monounsaturated.

Nutrient: Substances necessary to life that are found in food; carbohydrates, proteins, fats, vitamins, minerals, and water are nutrients.

Nutrition: The taking in and utilization of food to nourish the body.

Oral Hypoglycemic Agents: Many drugs, taken by mouth, which lower blood sugar; sometimes called **Antidiabetic Pills.**

Pancreas: A gland in the upper abdomen which secretes digestive enzymes into the intestine; it contains cells which produce two hormones called insulin and glucagon.

Polyunsaturated Fat: Fats found in vegetable oils which tend to lower blood cholesterol.

Protein: A major nutrient made up of amino acids that are necessary to maintain life; provides 4 calories per gram. The abbreviation for protein in our recipes is **PRO.**

Saccharin: An artificial sweetener that provides no carbohydrate or calories; read Chapter 20, "Sugar Substitutes."

Saturated Fat: Fats, mostly from animal foods, which tend to raise the level of blood cholesterol.

Sugar Alcohols: Sorbitol, Mannitol, and Xylitol; chemical substances that taste sweet but are more slowly absorbed by the body than sugars; in excess they act as a laxative; read Chapter 19, "The Great Sugar Masquerade."

Urinalysis: Chemical analysis of the urine.

Vitamins: Chemically organic substances found in food that are needed in very small amounts for normal body functions; includes Vitamins A, B Complex, C, D, E, and K.

II

The Diabetic Diet

Diet is the foundation of good control and management of diabetes mellitus. The restriction of certain foods and the moderation of total caloric intake are *musts* for all diabetics. In fact, in many cases of mild diabetes, especially in overweight people, the condition can be controlled by diet alone without oral medication or insulin. Generally, carbohydrate foods are limited and they also are spaced throughout the day to lessen the need for insulin production by the pancreas. Many diets for diabetics are modified by the doctor or diet counselor to meet other medical needs (such as fat or sodium restriction) that the individual may have.

All diabetic diets aim to provide all nutrients needed by the body. The well-planned diabetic diet is adequate in vitamins and minerals. Vitamin supplements should not be taken unless specifically prescribed by your physician. In fact, Vitamin C (ascorbic acid) in pill form may interfere with accuracy in testing of the urine for sugar.

Physicians have differing philosophies regarding the extent to which diet should be controlled. This depends somewhat on the kind of diabetes you may have, the severity of the condition, and your age when you became diabetic.

Some doctors believe entirely in the *weighed diet*. This is a diet in which all foods are weighed on a gram scale so that portion sizes and nutritive intake can be carefully controlled. Generally, this type of diet is used primarily for young diabetics and others whose diabetes is particularly difficult to control. Physicians who prefer the weighed diet believe that the stricter control results in less danger of complications, reduced symptoms, increased confidence in self-management, and general allover improvement in health and well-being.

Other doctors advocate much more permissive control depending upon the doctor's knowledge of the patient's willingness and ability to follow orders. With this philosophy the diabetic may be told to eat a *sugar-free diet* with moderate meals at regular mealtimes and to avoid sugar, cake, candy, honey, pastries, sweet rolls, sweet desserts, and regular soda pop. Often this type of diet is ordered for older diabetics who develop a very mild diabetes condition late in life, or for the individual who has limited ability to read or understand more complex instructions. These simplified instructions are more suitable for those who take oral hypoglycemic agents. Diabetics who require insulin do far better with a more precise diet and a more disciplined regime.

The *free diet* is prescribed by relatively few diabetologists for some children and teenagers. This diet is similar to the one just described, but the child or his parents are taught to give varying dosages of injected insulin depending upon the amount of sugar in the urine. Philosophically the idea is to let the child lead a more normal life with less dietary concern. But many in the medical world have questioned this free diet and insulin combination. There is some question as to whether or not it causes more early complications of the disease and more crisis care situations.

By far the most popular diet management of diabetes uses the *Food Exchange System* because it stresses moderate, regular food habits and allows the individual to choose from a wide variety of foods within his daily meal plan.

The Food Exchange System was developed in 1950 by a committee set up by the American Diabetes Association, Inc., the American Dietetic Association, and the Chronic Disease Program of the U.S. Public Health Service. The Food Exchanges underwent major revisions in 1976 on the basis of newer knowledge of nutrition and food composition. The updated Exchange Lists are concerned with total caloric intake and modification of fat intake as well as carbohydrate and protein values.

If you have been on a diabetic diet based on the old exchanges, you will see many differences. We hope that this book will help you to understand the new exchanges and to make an easier changeover to these new lists. Check with your own doctor to make sure that he approves of you using the new exchanges. If your doctor prefers that you stay on the old exchanges, and you have good control over your diabetes condition, then skip our lists and go on to other chapters of the book and the recipes. The nutritive values given for each recipe will still be useful to you.

Exchange? What Is That?

Before we tell you about the Food Exchange Lists, let's explain what is meant by the word *Exchange.* You know that you can trade or exchange 5 pennies for one 5¢ piece, or 10 dimes for a $1.00 bill. Right? OK. In the Food Exchanges within the same group, you may exchange 1 measurement or amount of 1 food for another food in that group. For example, look at List 3—Fruit Exchanges (Chapter 3). Your diet for breakfast may tell you to have 1 Fruit Exchange. So, you have been having ½ cup orange juice day after day. Want a change? Look over the list. Select the fruit you want in the serving amount given for 1 Fruit Exchange for that fruit and Exchange it for the ½ cup orange juice!

The Food Exchange System is based on a series of six Exchange Lists: Milk, Vegetables, Fruits, Breads, Meats, and Fats. Foods are grouped within each list on the basis of similar amounts of carbohydrate, protein, and fat. In order to do this, portion sizes must be identified for each food. For example, one Fruit Exchange (Yield: CHO 10 gm., PRO 0, FAT 0, Calories 40) is ½ cup of grapefruit juice but only ⅓ cup of pineapple juice. This is because pineapple juice has more carbohydrate (in this case sugar) than grapefruit juice. By varying portion sizes we come close to our goal of 10 grams of carbohydrate for each food on the Fruit List.

But keep in mind that there will be some surprises. Corn for example is a vegetable, but it appears on the Bread List. That is because corn is starchy and its carbohydrate value is much closer to bread than to most vegetables.

Each list has many foods. When your meal plan is determined by your doctor or diet counselor, the number of Exchanges for each meal will be planned. If, in the morning, for example, you are allowed 2 Bread Exchanges, you might choose ½ cup cooked oatmeal plus 1 piece of toast, *or* 1 cup of oatmeal, *or* 2 halves of a small toasted English Muffin. In other words, you may choose 2 different items from the Bread List or double the serving of one item to use up your two Bread Exchanges. This same concept applies to all other Exchange Lists too.

Your diet counselor will give you a meal plan, listing the Food Exchanges you are to eat at each meal. The meal plan will be based on your needs, your food habits, and any special dietary or medical problems that influence your individual needs. It is important to eat all of the food planned at each meal and to eat those meals at approximately the same time each day. No holdovers allowed! In other words, don't save up your Exchanges from one meal to eat at another time. Why? Because your body cannot properly use a big load of food at one time, and your medication may require food to work on at the time of the meal you have skipped.

The Exchange Lists here are reprinted from "Exchange Lists for Meal Planning" prepared by Committees of the American Diabetes Association, Inc., and the American Dietetic Association in cooperation with the National Institute of Arthritis, Metabolism and Digestive Diseases and the National Heart and Lung Institute, National Institutes of Health, Public Health Service, U.S. Department of Health, Education and Welfare. They are presented with the permission of both the American Diabetes Association, Inc., and the American Dietetic Association.

We have greatly expanded each of the lists by adding "Our Supplementary Exchanges," which include many items not in the standard teaching materials. For each added item we have checked the nutritive values with several sources especially with the newest tables of food composition and nutrient labeling on packages. Then we have calculated the proper portion size for one Exchange for each food.

At the end of each list you will find a discussion of how to use that list. The material in this section is a summary of many of the questions we have been asked in years of counseling individuals with diabetes mellitus. The discussion also includes a brief consideration of the nutrients contributed by each group. This was irresistible to us as nutrition educators.

And now the long awaited lists!

1

Milk Exchanges

For the diabetic diet, milk and milk products are included as List 1. Keep in mind that the word *exchange* may be considered as a trade. These foods in List 1 are related in Exchange values to 1 cup (8 ounces) skim milk, which supplies:

Carbohydrate: 12 grams
Protein: 8 grams
Fat: trace
Calories: 80

So, in reading List 1—Milk keep these values in mind. The measurement given for each food listed will yield these same nutritive values.

This List shows the kinds and amounts of milk or milk products to use for 1 Milk Exchange. Those which appear in **bold type** are **non-fat.** Low-Fat and Whole Milk contain saturated fat.

Non-Fat Fortified Milk

Skim or non-fat milk (liquid)	1 cup
Powdered (non-fat dry, before adding liquid)	⅓ cup
Canned, evaporated—skim milk	½ cup
Buttermilk made from skim milk	1 cup
Yogurt made from skim milk (plain, unflavored)	1 cup

Low-Fat Fortified Milk

1% fat fortified milk (omit ½ Fat Exchange)	1 cup
2% fat fortified milk (omit 1 Fat Exchange)	1 cup
Yogurt made from 2% fortified milk (plain, unflavored) (omit 1 Fat Exchange)	1 cup

Whole Milk (Omit 2 Fat Exchanges)

Whole Milk	1 cup
Canned, evaporated whole milk	½ cup
Buttermilk made from whole milk	1 cup
Yogurt made from whole milk (plain, unflavored)	1 cup

You will note that if you choose 1 cup of 1% fat fortified milk you must omit ½ Fat Exchange. To omit ½ Fat Exchange, first, look at List 6—Fat Exchanges (Chapter 6). Reduce the measurement of any choice on this list, for example, butter or margarine, allowed in the same meal by ½ teaspoon. To omit 1 Fat Exchange cut down by 1 teaspoon, and to omit 2 Fat Exchanges cut down by 2 teaspoons for that meal.

Although ice cream is a dairy product it is not included on the Milk Exchange List because it has too much carbohydrate and fat. Look on our Supplementary Bread List for ice milk; and on our Supplementary Fat List for ice cream.

Diabetics are advised not to use commercial flavored yogurts because so much carbohydrate has been added for sweetening. Use only the plain, unflavored yogurt. Turn to our recipes if you want to make delicious fruit-flavored yogurts (*see* Index).

The Milk Exchanges are our best sources of calcium, which is needed for bones and teeth, muscle contraction, and blood clotting. Milk also contributes high-quality protein. In addition, it is an excellent source of many other nutrients, especially phosphorus, riboflavin, and thiamin.

The Exchange List emphasis is on fortified milk which is available in your market. Most milk sold in the United States is fortified with Vitamin A (growth, eye functions, resistance to infection) and Vitamin D (for absorption and use of calcium). Milk has often been called a perfect food but it isn't. In fact, no one food provides all the nutrients we need. Milk, for example, is low in iron and Vitamin C (ascorbic acid) but its contributions are great in many other nutrients.

It is possible, but very difficult, to meet dietary needs for calcium and several of the vitamins and minerals if milk is not included in your daily meal plan. This is why most diet counselors include milk unless the diabetic patient shows a specific intolerance, an allergy, or a great dislike of milk. Some people who are physically intolerant of milk can eat fermented milk products such as yogurt or cheese. Ask your diet counselor to adjust your diet if you are unable to drink the milk in your plan. Most adult diets are planned with 2 cups of milk; children and teenagers usually drink 3 to 4 cups.

2

Vegetable Exchanges

In this list, List 2—Vegetable Exchanges, the nutritive value of each vegetable is similar. To make it easier to remember, the values have been averaged so that one serving of any vegetable in this list (fresh, frozen, or canned) supplies:

Carbohydrate: 5 grams
Protein: 2 grams
Fat: 0
Calories: 28

This List shows the kinds of **vegetables** to use for 1 Vegetable Exchange. 1 Exchange is **½ cup.**

Asparagus
Bean Sprouts
Beets
Broccoli
Brussels Sprouts
Cabbage
Carrots
Cauliflower
Celery
Cucumbers
Eggplant
Green Pepper

Greens:
  Beet
  Chards
  Collards
  Dandelion
  Kale
  Mustard
  Spinach
  Turnip
Mushrooms
Okra
Onions

Rhubarb
Rutabaga
Sauerkraut
String Beans, Green or Yellow
Summer Squash

Tomatoes
Tomato Juice
Turnips
Vegetable Juice Cocktail
Zucchini

The following **raw vegetables** may be used as desired:

Chicory
Chinese Cabbage
Endive
Escarole

Lettuce
Parsley
Radishes
Watercress

Starchy Vegetables are found in the Bread Exchange List.

Our Supplementary Vegetable List

One Vegetable Exchange is ½ cup of a vegetable, measured cooked or raw (unless another measure is indicated).

Artichoke, Globe, 1 medium
Asparagus, 5 large or 8
    small spears
Bamboo Shoots
Beans, Italian, Pole or Wax
Broccoli, 1 whole small stalk
Cabbage, Green or Red
Carrots, 1 medium whole
Green Onions, Scallions
Kohlrabi
Leeks, 2 medium

Pea Pods, including Chinese
Pimiento, whole
Red Peppers, cooked
Tomatoes, fresh, whole, 1
    medium
Tomatoes, Cherry, about 6
Tomatoes, cooked or canned
Tomato Catsup, 2 tablespoons
Tomato Paste, 2 tablespoons
Tomato Sauce
Water Chestnuts, canned, about
    6 whole

These raw vegetables may be used as desired. Up to 2 cups of any one of the following vegetables may be counted as 1 Vegetable Exchange:

Celantro (Coriander)
Green Pepper, raw

Red Pepper, raw
Spinach, raw

Starchy vegetables are included in List 4—Breads and Cereals (Chapter 4), because their carbohydrate contents are so much higher than most vegetables and are similar to the amounts of carbohydrates in breads.

A small amount of a vegetable used as a seasoning or garnish need not be counted as a vegetable. For example, a slice of tomato or onion on a sandwich can be included without using up a Vegetable Exchange. We interpret "The following raw vegetables to be used as desired" to mean that you may eat more than the ½ cup portion indicated for 1 Vegetable Exchange. We calculated that it would be safe to eat up to about 2 cups of these vegetables and only count one Vegetable Exchange. Vegetables on these lists may be eaten alone or mixed. For example, a salad containing lettuce, celery, cucumbers, and green peppers counts as only 1 Vegetable Exchange if you eat no more than 2 cups, which is a large salad. We assume that there will be far more lettuce than the other vegetables.

We are very fortunate here in America to have such a wide choice of vegetables—fresh, canned, frozen, and dried. Whether you grow your own, buy from a market gardener, or buy from a supermarket, be guided by this list of Vegetable Exchanges for the diabetic. They add color and texture to your meals as well as providing several important nutrients.

Dark green and deep yellow vegetables are particularly rich sources of carotene, which changes in our bodies to Vitamin A. The deeper the color of the vegetable the better the source. For example, spinach is a better source of this nutrient, carotene, than is iceberg lettuce. Vitamin A promotes growth, is needed for good vision, promotes resistance to infection, and maintains skin tone.

Brussels sprouts, peppers, broccoli, cabbage, and tomatoes are excellent sources of Vitamin C. Vegetables are also good sources of several vitamins of the B Complex and a few minerals, and they are a most popular source of dietary fiber. So, as you fill up on low-calorie vegetables, know that they are nutritious as well as delicious!

3

Fruit Exchanges

List 3—Fruit Exchanges includes choices from one of our most popular food groups. Because the nutritive values of individual fruits vary so widely there can be no allover rule as to the amount or measurement per serving. Therefore, this list gives the measured amounts or sizes of each fruit. In each case, however, each measurement or amount is for a single fresh, frozen, canned (waterpack), or dried fruit, without the addition of sugar in any form. Each serving or Exchange of fruit listed here supplies:

Carbohydrate: 10 grams
Protein: 0
Fat: 0
Calories: 40

This List shows the kinds and amounts of **fruits** to use for 1 Fruit Exchange.

Apple	1 small	**Blueberries**	½ cup
Apple Juice	⅓ cup	**Raspberries**	½ cup
Applesauce (unsweetened)	½ cup	**Strawberries**	¾ cup
Apricots, fresh	2 medium	**Cherries**	10 large
Apricots, dried	4 halves	**Cider**	⅓ cup
Banana	½ small	**Cranberries** may be	
Berries		used as desired if	
Blackberries	½ cup	no sugar is added.	

Dates	2	Orange	1 small
Figs, fresh	1	Orange Juice	½ cup
Figs, dried	1	Papaya	¾ cup
Grapefruit	½	Peach	1 medium
Grapefruit Juice	½ cup	Pear	1 small
Grapes	12	Persimmon, native	1 medium
Grape Juice	¼ cup	Pineapple	½ cup
Mango	½ small	Pineapple Juice	⅓ cup
Melon		Plums	2 medium
Cantaloupe	¼ small	Prunes	2 medium
Honeydew	⅛ medium	Prune Juice	¼ cup
Watermelon	1 cup	Raisins	2 tablespoons
Nectarine	1 small	Tangerine	1 medium

Our Supplementary Fruit List

Apple Cider, unsweetened	⅓ cup
Bananas, sliced	⅓ cup
Berries	
Gooseberries	⅔ cup
Loganberries	½ cup
Mulberries	½ cup
Cherries, Maraschino	4
Cherries, sour red	½ cup
Currants, dried	1 tablespoon
Figs, canned	⅓ cup
Fruit Cocktail, unsweetened	½ cup
Grapefruit Segments	½ cup
Grapefruit Instant Breakfast Drink, liquid	⅓ cup
Grapes, small	20
Grape Instant Breakfast Drink, Liquid	⅓ cup
Ground Cherries	½ cup

Guava	1 small
Jicama	1
Kumquats	4 medium
Lemon, whole	1 large
Lemon Juice	½ cup
Limes	2
Lime Juice	½ cup
Loquats	6
Lychees, fresh or dried	7
Mango, diced or sliced	⅓ cup
Melon, Casaba	¹⁄₁₀
Melon Balls or Cubes	¾ cup
Mixed Fresh Fruits, unsweetened	½ cup
Nectars (Apricot, Peach, Pear), unsweetened	⅓
Orange Segments, fresh	½ cup
Papaya, 5 inches long	⅓
Peaches, dried	2 small halves
Pears, sliced or cubed	⅓ cup
Pears, dried	½
Pineapple, sliced, canned in pineapple juice	1 slice plus 2 tablespoons juice
Pineapple, sliced, canned in pineapple juice	2 slices, drained
Pineapple Tidbits or Chunks	⅓ cup
Pomegranate, medium	⅓
Raisins	½ ounce package
Tang Instant Breakfast Drink, liquid	⅓ cup
Tangelos	1 medium
Tangerine Juice, unsweetened	⅓ cup

Fresh fruits in season are generally the best choice for both flavor and texture. Whether you choose frozen, dried, or canned fruits there should be no sugar added. Read Chapter 19, "The Great Sugar Masquerade," for an explanation of the names of various sugars which may be added in the processing of fruit.

Canned fruits are quite popular, especially in the wintertime when fewer fresh fruits are available. But canned fruits have widely varying carbohydrate content depending on the liquid used in the canning process. Diabetics should not use any fruit canned in regular syrup—light, medium, or heavy. Before the introduction of water- and juice-packed fruits, diabetics were told to use these fruits but to wash off the syrup. Well, it doesn't work! A fruit that sits for months in a heavy sugar syrup absorbs much of that sugar throughout the fruit. If you were to use syrup-packed canned fruit that was washed, you would have to cut your serving size at least in half to have the correct carbohydrate value.

Instead, we suggest that you buy water-packed fruits with or without added artificial sweetener. Our portions for fruit exchanges for canned fruits are based on water-packed fruits unless otherwise indicated.

Kay has a trick she always uses to make water-packed fruits more delicious. Carefully, she drains the fruit, saving the liquid. She transfers the fruit to a glass jar. To the drained liquid she adds 1 to 2 teaspoons lemon juice and just enough artificial sweetener to make it pleasant and tasty. When well mixed, she pours this back on top of the fruit, covers the jar, and stores it in the refrigerator for 24 hours. Presto! The fruit has more fruity flavor and even the liquid tastes good.

An acceptable alternative is the even more flavorful juice-packed fruit, which has recently become widely available. Pineapple has been canned in unsweetened pineapple juice for years, but lately pears, peaches, and other fruits, packed in unsweetened white grape juice or unsweetened nectar, are available in supermarkets. Of course the juice has its own carbohydrate value. Read our suggestions on "How to Read a Label" (Chapter 17), then read carefully the nutritive values on the canned fruits. Drain the juice and measure it to be counted as an additional Fruit Exchange *or* reduce the portion size of the fruit. For example, if you are using water-packed or fresh fruit cocktail, your portion for 1 Fruit Exchange is ½ cup. But if you use juice-packed fruit cocktail reduce the portion size to ⅓ cup for 1 Fruit Exchange. This is because the actual carbohydrate value is 10 grams for water-packed fruit, versus 14 grams for the same ½ cup portion of juice-packed fruit. By reducing the portion size you will still be using 1 Fruit Exchange. Another example is our old standby pineapple. A serving is 2 rings without any juice from juice-packed pineapple or 1 ring plus 2 tablespoons of the juice.

Fruits are valuable sources of vitamins, minerals, and fiber. Most of us get almost all of the Vitamin C (ascorbic acid) that we need every day from this food group. Citrus fruits, such as oranges, grapefruits, tangerines, and lemons are the best food sources. Most Americans get their Vitamin C at breakfast, but other meals may also include rich Vitamin C sources such as strawberries, mangoes, cantaloupe, or honeydew melon. Vitamin C is necessary for the formation of healthy connective tissue and bones. It also has other important functions in the body. Early symptoms of insufficient Vitamin C in the diet include bleeding gums and the tendency to bruise easily.

The functions of Vitamin A are described in Chapter 2, "Vegetable Exchanges." Excellent fruit sources include fruits which are orange in color—apricots, mangoes, cantaloupe, nectarines, yellow peaches, and persimmons. All of these fruits also yield the mineral, potassium. Oranges, bananas, and dried fruits join the list to give us potassium. Potassium is very necessary in maintaining good cellular metabolic reactions, the nervous system, and energy metabolism.

4

Bread Exchanges

Bread, cereals, starchy vegetables, and some prepared foods are all included in List 4. One Bread Exchange yields:

Carbohydrate: 15 grams
Protein: 2 grams
Fat: 0
Calories: 68

Many brand names are used in Our Supplementary Bread List. We remind you that the use of brand names is not a product endorsement by the publisher or the authors. Brand names are used only so that you will know what product we are identifying and you may then substitute a similar type of product using the same measure.

This List shows the kinds and amounts of **Breads, Cereals, Starchy Vegetables** and Prepared Foods to use for one Bread Exchange. Those which appear in **bold type** are **low-fat**.

Bread

White (including French and Italian)	1 slice
Whole Wheat	1 slice
Rye or Pumpernickel	1 slice
Raisin	1 slice

Bagel, small	½
English Muffin, small	½
Plain Roll, bread	1
Frankfurter Roll	½
Hamburger Bun	½
Dried Bread Crumbs	3 tablespoons
Tortilla, 6 inches (not fried)	1

Cereal

Bran Flakes	½ cup
Other ready-to-eat unsweetened Cereal	¾ cup
Puffed Cereal (unfrosted)	1 cup
Cereal (cooked)	½ cup
Grits (cooked)	½ cup
Rice or Barley (cooked)	½ cup
Pasta (cooked) Spaghetti, Noodles, Macaroni	½ cup
Popcorn (popped, no fat added)	3 cups
Cornmeal (dry)	2 tablespoons
Flour	2½ tablespoons
Wheat Germ	¼ cup

Crackers

Arrowroot	3
Graham, 2½-inch square	2
Matzoth, 4-inch by 6-inch	½
Oyster	20
Pretzels, 3⅛-inch long by ⅛-inch diameter	25
Rye Wafers, 2-inch by 3½-inch	3
Saltines	6
Soda, 2½-inch square	4

Dried Beans, Peas and Lentils

Beans, Peas, Lentils (dried and cooked)	½ cup
Baked Beans, no pork (canned)	¼ cup

Starchy Vegetables

Corn	⅓ cup
Corn on Cob	1 small
Lima Beans	½ cup
Parsnips	⅔ cup
Peas, Green (canned or frozen)	½ cup
Potato, White	1 small
Potato (mashed)	½ cup
Pumpkin	¾ cup
Winter Squash, Acorn or Butternut	½ cup
Yam or Sweet Potato	¼ cup

Prepared Foods

Biscuit 2-inch diameter (omit 1 Fat Exchange)	1
Corn Bread, 2-inch by 2-inch by 1-inch (omit 1 Fat Exchange)	1
Corn Muffin, 2-inch diameter (omit 1 Fat Exchange)	1
Crackers, round butter type (omit 1 Fat Exchange)	5
Muffin, plain small (omit 1 Fat Exchange)	1
Potatoes, French Fried, length 2-inch to 3½-inch (omit 1 Fat Exchange)	8
Potato or Corn Chips (omit 2 Fat Exchanges)	15
Pancake, 5-inch by ½-inch (omit 1 Fat Exchange)	1
Waffle, 5-inch by ½-inch (omit 1 Fat Exchange)	1

Our Supplementary Bread List

BREAD

Bialy Roll	1
Boston Brown Bread (3-inch diameter, ½-inch thick)	1 slice
Bread Cubes or Plain Croutons	1 cup
Bread Sticks (8 inches long, ½-inch diameter)	2 sticks
Bread Sticks (4 inches long, ¼-inch diameter)	6 sticks

Cracked or Sprouted Wheat Bread	1 slice
Party Rye, small rounds	3 to 4 slices
Pita, Syrian Bread	¼ slice
Very Thin Sliced Bread, White or Dark	1½ slices

CEREALS AND GRAINS

DO NOT use sugar or honey coated cereals. DO
  NOT use granola type cereals.

Barley (uncooked)	1½ tablespoons
Bran Cereals, ready to eat	½ cup
Buckwheat, Kasha (cooked)	½ cup
Bulgar (uncooked)	2 tablespoons
Cornflake Crumbs	3 tablespoons
Cornstarch	2 tablespoons
Farfel (uncooked)	3 tablespoons
Grapenuts	3 tablespoons
Rice, cooked, measured hot	⅓ cup
Shredded Wheat Biscuit, unsweetened	1 biscuit

CRACKERS

Cheese-Nips (omit 1 Fat Exchange)	20
Cheese Tid-Bits (omit 1 Fat Exchange)	28
Chicken In A Biscuit (omit 1 Fat Exchange)	10
Chippers (omit 1 Fat Exchange)	7
Cracker Meal	2½ tablespoons
Holland Rusks	1½ biscuits
Matzoth (6-inch round)	1
Melba Toast, rectangles	5
Melba Toast, rounds	8
Pretzels, Dutch	1
Pretzels, Three-Ring	6
Pretzel Rods (7½ inches long)	1½
Pretzels, Veri-Thin	65
Ritz-Cheese (omit 1 Fat Exchange)	7
Ritz Crackers (omit 1 Fat Exchange)	7
Rye Thins (omit 1 Fat Exchange)	10
Sociables (omit 1 Fat Exchange)	12
Triangle Thins	15
Triscuits	5
Uneeda Biscuit	4
Waverly Wafers	6
Wheat Thins	12
Zwieback Toast	3 pieces

Our Supplementary Bread List (continued)

DRIED BEANS, PEAS AND LENTILS

Chick Peas, Garbanzo Beans, cooked	¼ cup
Lima Beans, dried and cooked	⅓ cup

Actually, these dried beans and peas are protein as well as carbohydrate sources. For people who eat dried beans occasionally this is not a major concern. But if you eat lots of dried beans and peas you should discuss this with your diet counselor and the diet counselor will adjust your allowed Meat Exchanges to include these protein values.

STARCHY VEGETABLES

Boniato, boiled	½ cup
Chayote, boiled	½ cup
Malanga, boiled	½ cup
Ñame, boiled	½ cup
Potato, Hash Browns (omit 1 Fat Exchange)	¼ cup
Potato Flakes (dry)	⅓ cup
Potato, Mashed, made from flakes with fat as directed (omit 1 Fat Exchange)	½ cup
Salsify, Oyster Plant	¾ cup
Yautia, boiled	½ cup
Yucca, boiled	½ cup

Use the following only with the permission of your doctor or diet counselor and after carefully reading "About Cookies and Crackers," which follows.

PREPARED FOODS

Angel Food Cake, no frosting	1½-inch cube
Animal Crackers, Barnums	7
Arrowroot Cookies	4
Brown Edge Wafer Cookies (omit ½ Fat Exchange)	3
Cheese Puffs (omit 2 Fat Exchanges)	1 cup
Chocolate Chip Cookies, 1¾ inches diameter (omit 1 Fat Exchange)	3

Chow Mein Noodles (omit 1 Fat Exchange)	½ cup
Cinnamon Crisps, broken on line	4
Doughnut, plain, cake type	1 small
Fig Bar	1
Fig Newton Cake	1½
Gingersnaps	3
Graham Cracker Crumbs	¼ cup
Ice Cream Cone, Wafer type (not Sugar Cone)	2
Ice Milk, Vanilla, soft-style (omit ½ **Fat** Exchange)	⅓ cup
Ice Milk, Vanilla, hard type (omit ½ Fat Exchange)	½ cup
Ladyfingers	1 large, 2 small
Lorna Doone Shortbread Cookies (omit 1 Fat Exchange)	3
Malted Powder, plain dry	2 tablespoons
Onion Rings, frozen (omit 2 Fat Exchanges)	⅕ of 10-ounce package
Oreo Creme Sandwich, not with extra filling (omit 1 Fat Exchange)	2
Potato Stix, Shoestring Potatoes (omit 2 Fat Exchanges)	¾ cup
Social Tea Biscuits, plain	4
Sponge Cake, no frosting	1½-inch cube
Sugar Wafers (omit 1 Fat Exchange)	6
Tater-Tots, Potato Puffs (omit 1½ Fat Exchanges)	½ cup
Vanilla Wafers (omit ½ Fat Exchange)	5

In addition to the 1 Bread Exchange to be used for each of the above items, many of them also direct you to omit ½, 1, or 2 Fat Exchanges. To omit 1 Fat Exchange, look at List 6—Fat Exchanges. Reduce your choices from that list, for example butter or margarine, allowed in the same meal by 1 teaspoon. Do not use up more Fat Exchanges for any one meal than your diet plan allows.

About Cookies and Crackers

Some of you may question the listing of many cookies and crackers in Our Supplementary List. We know that diabetics want to eat regular, commercial products. And we want them to, as much as can be allowed, so that they can enjoy the same things the family does. Special dietetic products fool people in that they are often not lower in nutritive values than the regular ones, their labels are very misleading, and they cost more. Our own extensive test-kitchen work has proved to us that baked, sweet-flavor cookies require a sweetener, and they cannot be made successfully by using the presently available artificial sweeteners. Therefore, we have included very few cookie recipes among our recipes, and even those have some sugar. We believe that some commercial products of known food composition can be used occasionally by some diabetics. We remind you that these all contain one or more types of sugar, and therefore caution you to use moderation in eating them, whether for snacks or regular meals. Discuss these products with your own physician or diet counselor before adding them to your meal plan. The Food Exchanges listed for each cookie or cracker are based on careful reference to the most recent nutritive values.

Please don't try to use Aunt Tillie's home recipe for a cookie, in the same portion stated in this list. It is not a fair exchange. Aunt Tillie's recipe may have more butter or sugar or may be twice the size of the commercial product. If you must share Aunt Tillie's bounty, take the recipe to your diet counselor who can calculate nutritive values and Exchange values for you. Sorry, Aunt Tillie!

The Bread List contains a wide variety of foods. Whole grain and enriched breads and cereals, wheat germ, bran products, and dried beans and peas are good sources of iron (which carries oxygen to cells and performs other metabolic functions) and thiamin (for metabolic activity in every cell of the body). This group also contributes necessary potassium and folacin (a vitamin of the B Complex).

Whole grain, wheat germ, dried beans and peas, and especially bran products have a great deal of fiber—much more than foods made from refined flour. Fiber has recently become a popular nutrient. We used to think of fiber as just a waste product. Now we know that fiber not only adds bulk to our diet but it has been suggested by researchers that diets too low in fiber increase the risk of getting certain bowel cancers, gastrointestinal disorders, and even coronary heart disease. Yet, great excesses of fiber seem to interfere with the absorption of calcium and zinc. Unless you have other major problems, diabetics need not be concerned about excesses of fiber. Your allotted Exchanges provide enough fiber for the positive activities of digestion but not nearly enough to interfere with mineral utilization. Do try to choose fiber foods, such as whole grain cereals and breads, bran products, dried fruits, nuts, and raw vegetables, each day.

5

Meat Exchanges

The meat family in List 5—Meat Exchanges includes meats, fish, poultry, eggs, cheese, peanut butter, and dried peas and beans. This is because all of these foods are rich sources of protein. This big group is subdivided into three smaller groups according to the fat content of each food. The first group is called *LEAN MEATS;* the second group is called *MEDIUM-FAT MEATS;* the third group is called *HIGH-FAT MEATS.*

For each food, the 1-ounce portion nutritive values are based on the cooked food with all separable fats removed. In other words, take your *cooked* meat, remove separable fat and bones, and weigh the edible, remaining meat. If you are allowed 3 Meat Exchanges at dinner, for example, you may weigh out a 3-ounce portion.

Our Supplementary Meat Lists are all based upon information provided by the National Livestock and Meat Board from their publications and from discussions with them. All of the Supplementary Meat Lists include common names you may see in your grocery store or meat market. Some are actually the same cut of meat as in the original lists but have different names. These added names will help you to identify the cuts you can choose. Also, many restaurants use a number of these names to describe their meat selections.

Determining the fat content of each meat cut posed special problems because the 1976 Exchange List did not always agree with our advice from the National Livestock and Meat Board. We have tried to make the Supplementary Lists as accurate as possible within the framework provided by the original Lists.

Lean Meats

All protein foods listed here are low in fat. One Exchange of any one of these foods, cooked, yields:

Carbohydrate: 0
Protein: 7 grams
Fat: 3 grams
Calories: 55

All foods listed here are recommended for low-fat, fat-modified, or low-cholesterol diets.

This List shows the kinds and amounts of **Lean Meat** and other Protein-Rich Foods to use for 1 Low-Fat Meat Exchange.

Beef:	**Baby Beef (very lean), Chipped Beef, Chuck, Flank Steak, Tenderloin, Plate Ribs, Plate Skirt Steak, Round (bottom, top), All cuts Rump, Spare Ribs, Tripe**	1 ounce
Lamb:	**Leg, Rib, Sirloin, Loin (roast and chops), Shank, Shoulder**	1 ounce
Pork:	**Leg (Whole Rump, Center Shank), Ham, Smoked (center slices)**	1 ounce
Veal:	**Leg, Loin, Rib, Shank, Shoulder, Cutlets**	1 ounce
Poultry:	**Meat without skin of Chicken, Turkey, Cornish Hen, Guinea Hen, Pheasant**	1 ounce
Fish:	**Any fresh or frozen**	1 ounce
	Canned Salmon, Tuna, Mackerel, Crab, Lobster	¼ cup
	Clams, Oysters, Scallops, Shrimp	5 or 1 ounce
	Sardines, drained	3

Cheeses containing less than 5% butterfat	1 ounce
Cottage Cheese, Dry and 2% butterfat	¼ cup
Dried Beans and Peas (omit 1 Bread Exchange)	½ cup

Our Supplementary Lean Meat List

BEEF

Braciole Steak
Beef Shanks
Beef Stroganoff
Cap Meat Rolled
Crescent Roast
Cubed Flank Steak
Dried Chipped Beef
Eye of Round Roast or Steak
Family Steak
Filet Mignon
Flank Steak Filet
Flip Steaks, Sandwich Steaks
Jewish Tenderloin
Kabob Cubes

Loin Steak, boneless
London Broil
London Grill Steak
Pepper Steak
Rolled Plate
Round Steak
Rump Roast
Rump Steak
Skirt Steak
Stew Beef, trimmed of separable fat
Tenderloin tips
Top Round Roast
Very Lean Ground Round,
    90% lean
Very Lean Ground Sirloin, 90% lean

LAMB

Chops, Rib, or Shoulder,
    well trimmed
Crown Roast of Lamb,
    well trimmed
Cushion Roast of Lamb
Lamb Cubes, lean
Lamb Neck for stew

Lamb Steaks
Rack of Lamb, well trimmed
Shish Kebob
Shoulder Roast
Sirloin Roast
Square-cut Shoulder

CHEESE

2% low-fat cottage cheese
1% low-fat cottage cheese

Light n' Lively
Lite-Line
Tastee Loaf

BEANS

Soybean Curd, Tofu—3 ounces

Medium-Fat Meats

All of the protein foods listed here are moderate in fat. One Exchange of any one of these foods, cooked, yields:

Carbohydrate: 0
Protein: 7 grams
Fat: 5.5 grams
Calories: 77

This is equivalent to one Lean Meat plus ½ Fat Exchange. Only peanut butter is recommended for those on fat-modified, low-cholesterol diets.

This List shows the kinds and amounts of Medium-Fat Meat and other Protein-Rich Foods to use for 1 Medium-Fat Meat Exchange.

Beef:	Ground (15% fat), Corned Beef (canned), Rib Eye, Round (ground commercial)	1 ounce
Pork:	Loin (all cuts Tenderloin), Shoulder Arm (picnic), Shoulder Blade, Boston Butt, Canadian Bacon, Boiled Ham	1 ounce
	Liver, Heart, Kidney, Sweetbreads (these are high in cholesterol)	1 ounce
	Cottage Cheese, cream-style	¼ cup
	Cheese: Mozzarella, Ricotta, Farmer's cheese,	1 ounce
	Neufchatel, Parmesan	3 tablespoons
	Egg (high in cholesterol)	1
	Peanut Butter (omit 2 additional Fat Exchanges)	2 tablespoons

Our Supplementary Medium-Fat Meat List

Each ounce of boneless, cooked meat equals 1 Medium-Fat Meat Exchange *or* 1 Lean Meat Exchange plus ½ Fat Exchange. **Trim off all separable fat before weighing meat.**

BEEF

Barbecue Chuck Steak
Blade Steak
Boneless Chuck Roast, well trimmed

Boneless English Cut Roast
Boston Cut Roast
California Steak or Roast

Cross-cut Rib Roast
Delmonico Steak or Roast
Eye of Chuck Roast
Honey Cut Roast
Kansas City Steak
New York Strip Steak
Porterhouse Steak

Puff Roast
Shoulder Steak
Sirloin Steak or Roast
Sirloin Tip Roast
T-Bone Steak
Triangle Roast

PORK

Boneless Pork Cubes
Boneless Pork Loin Roast
Breakfast Pork Chops
Butterfly Pork Chops
Canadian Bacon, Back Bacon
Chipped Ham
Crown Roast of Pork

Fresh Pork Butt
Pork Cutlets
Pork Loin Roast
Pork Sirloin Chops
Pork Tenderloin
Smoked Pork Chops or
  Roast

VEAL

Veal Frankfurters
Veal Riblets

FISH

Anchovy Fillets, drained—9
Caviar, Fish Roe—1 ounce
Eel, American

Sablefish
Salmon, Chinook

CHEESE

American Cheese Spread
Kraft Golden Image Singles (high in polyunsaturated fats)
Monterey Jack
Velveeta Cheese

High-Fat Meats

All of these foods are high in fat; in fact, they have even more fat than protein! One ounce of cooked meat, trimmed of all separable fat and bone, yields:

Carbohydrate: 0
Protein: 7 grams
Fat: 8 grams
Calories: 100

One High-Fat Meat Exchange is equivalent to 1 Lean Meat Exchange plus 1 Fat Exchange. These foods are *not* recommended for low-fat, fat-modified or low-cholesterol diets.

This list shows the kinds and amounts of High-Fat Meat and other Protein-Rich Foods to use for one High-Fat Meat Exchange.

Beef:	Brisket, Corned Beef (Brisket), Ground Beef (more than 20% fat), Hamburger (commercial), Chuck (ground commercial), Roasts (Rib), Steaks (Club and Rib)	1 ounce
Lamb:	Breast	1 ounce
Pork:	Spare Ribs, Loin (Back Ribs), Pork (ground), Country-style Ham, Deviled Ham	1 ounce
Veal:	Breast	1 ounce
Poultry:	Capon, Duck (domestic), Goose	1 ounce
Cheese:	Cheddar Types	1 ounce
Cold Cuts		4½-inch-by-⅛-inch slice
Frankfurter		1 small or ½ medium

Our Supplementary High-Fat Meat List

Each ounce of cooked meat should be trimmed of bone and all separable fat. Because these meats are so high in fat you should be particularly careful to trim off excess fat before weighing out the diabetic's portion of meat. You will be surprised at finding so little edible meat on many of these cuts. Mary bought a 2¾-pound pot roast and, after it was cooked, it weighed out to less than 1 pound of lean cooked meat!

BEEF
Arm Pot Roast and Steaks
Barbecue Ribs
Beef Tongue
Blade-cut Chuck Roast
Chuck Pot Roast
Chuck Short Ribs
Chuck Stew Beef
Flanken
Round Bone Pot Roast
Short Ribs
Yankee Pot Roast

LAMB
Riblets

PORK
Barbecue Ribs
Country Ribs
Fresh Pork Belly
Fresh Side of Pork
Hock, Smoked Hock
Pig's Feet
Pork Shanks
Pork Tails
Smoked Pork Ribs

CHEESE
Black Diamond
Blue
Brick
Brie
Camembert
Caraway
Cheshire
Colby
Edam
Feta
Fontina
Gjetost (CHO 12 gm.)
Gouda
Gruyere
Muenster
Port Salut
Provolone
Romano
Roquefort
Swiss
Tilset
Pasteurized Process:
 American
 Pimiento
 Swiss
 American Cheese Food
 Swiss Cheese Food
 Cold Pack American
  Cheese Food

Kraft Golden Image Imitation Cheddar (high in polyunsaturated fats)
Kraft Golden Image Imitation Colby (high in polyunsaturated fats)
Limburger

FRANKFURTERS
Cocktail Weiners—3
Small Vienna Sausages—3

Diet counselors are not in complete agreement as to how the 3 Meat Lists are to be calculated into individualized meal plans. Some counselors calculate strictly on the basis of Lean Meats and then there are extra fats available which may be used for food from the Fat Exchange List or from Medium-Fat or High-Fat Meats. Others tell their patients to choose primarily Lean Meats but a few Medium-Fat or High-Fat Meats throughout the week, and then the Meal Plan is calculated on the basis of a somewhat higher fat value than the 3 grams of a Lean Meat. Your diet counselor will give you additional explanation as to which of the meat values was used in planning your meals. Our recipes give both the nutritive values and the translation of that information into the correct Exchanges.

The Meat Group provides many important nutrients. All foods from the Meat Lists supply protein, which helps to form and maintain all cells of the body. Protein also provides calories and each gram of protein yields 4 calories. Although proteins and carbohydrates are used differently in the body, an excess of protein can be converted to glucose, so it is wise to weigh your portions of protein foods.

Iron carries oxygen to the cells and is necessary for blood formation. Many women do not get enough of this mineral and they develop *iron-deficiency anemia*. Iron is found in liver, red meats, egg yolk, dried peas, and beans. Cooking in an old-fashioned black cast-iron pot or skillet, one not coated with enamel, can also increase the iron content of the diet. Also necessary for proper blood formation and the prevention of another type of anemia is Vitamin B_{12}, which is found only in foods of animal origin. Most foods of the Meat Group help meet dietary needs for B_{12}, but vegetarians and others who select vegetable choices from the Meat Group (dried beans, peas, peanut butter, etc.) may need dietary supplements.

Zinc is a mineral needed in tiny amounts. Scientists have found that it combines with insulin for proper storage of the hormone. Zinc has also been found to influence our ability to taste foods and is necessary for metabolism. This nutrient is provided by meats, poultry, liver, seafood, eggs, and dried peas. Potassium helps maintain the acid-base balance of the body and is necessary for nerve and muscle activity, glycogen formation, and protein usage.

Meats, dried peas and beans, and peanut butter supply potassium, as do many fruits and vegetables.

Specific foods of the Meat Group are excellent sources of other nutrients. Lean pork supplies considerable amounts of thiamin; seafoods supply iodine, which is also available to us through the use of iodized salt; the soft edible bones of canned tuna, salmon, and sardines provide calcium, although we get most of the calcium in our diet from the Milk Group. And then there is liver—rich in Vitamin A and at least 12 other nutrients! But this nutrient package is also rich in cholesterol and is a poor choice if you have been advised to limit your intake of dietary cholesterol.

6

Fat Exchanges

Although the foods listed in List 6—Fats are not as colorful as other types of foods, they have a definite place in many popular methods of cooking, and frequently they complement the flavor of other foods. All fats are concentrated in calories, whether they are in solid, whipped, or liquid form. For this reason we caution you to measure them accurately. It's so easy to get too generous! Right now, it is important for you to know that each of the foods listed here, in the measurement or amount given, yields:

Carbohydrate: 0
Protein: 0
Fat: 5 grams
Calories: 45

This List shows the kinds and amounts of Fat-Containing Foods to use for 1 Fat Exchange. To plan a diet low in Saturated Fat select only those Exchanges which appear in **bold type.** They are **Polyunsaturated.**

Margarine, soft, tub, or stick*	1 teaspoon
Avocado (4 inches in diameter)**	⅛
Oil: Corn, Cottonseed, Safflower, Soy, Sunflower	1 teaspoon
Oil, Olive**	1 teaspoon
Oil, Peanut**	1 teaspoon
Olives**	5 small
Almonds**	10 whole
Pecans**	2 large whole
Peanuts**	
Spanish	20 whole
Virginia	10 whole
Walnuts	6 small
Nuts, other**	6 small
Margarine, regular stick	1 teaspoon
Butter	1 teaspoon
Bacon fat	1 teaspoon
Bacon, crisp	1 strip
Cream, light	2 tablespoons
Cream, sour	2 tablespoons
Cream, heavy	1 tablespoon
Cream Cheese	1 tablespoon
French dressing***	1 tablespoon
Italian dressing***	1 tablespoon
Lard	1 teaspoon
Mayonnaise***	1 teaspoon
Salad dressing, mayonnaise type***	2 teaspoons
Salt pork	¾ inch cube

* Made with corn, cottonseed, safflower, soy, or sunflower oil only.
** Fat content is primarily monounsaturated.
*** If made with corn, cottonseed, safflower, soy, or sunflower oil can be used on fat-modified diet.

Our Supplementary Fat List

Most fats are mixtures of all three types of fatty acids but the type in the greatest amount is indicated as characteristic of that food. Soft margarines made from corn or safflower oil have more polyunsaturated fatty acids than hard margarine. We have marked most foods with the type of fatty acids they contain the most of: (P) primarily polyunsaturated; (M) primarily monounsaturated; (S) primarily saturated.

Anchiote, prepared (S)	2 teaspoons
Avocado, 4 inches (M)	⅛
Avocado, mashed (M)	2 tablespoons
Bacon, thick sliced (S)	½ strip, crisp
Bleu Cheese, Roquefort Dressing,	
commercial (P)	2 teaspoons
Butter Pat, 1¼ inch by ⅓ inch (S)	1½ pats
Butter, whipped (S)	2 teaspoons
Chicken Fat (M)	1 teaspoon
Chitterlings, fried (S)	1 tablespoon
Cracklins, Pork (S)	1 rounded teaspoon
Ice Cream, plain Vanilla 10% fat	
(omit 1 Bread Exchange) (S)	½ cup
Margarine Pat, 1¼ inch by ⅓ inch (M)	1½ pats
Margarine, whipped (M)	1½ teaspoons
Pork Sausage Patty, 1 ounce raw, cooked,	
and drained	
(omit ½ High-Fat Meat) (S)	1
Sofrito (S)	2 teaspoons
Tartar Sauce (P)	2 teaspoons
Thousand Island or Russian Dressing,	
commercial (P)	2 teaspoons

SHELLED NUTS

Almonds, chopped (M)	1 tablespoon
Brazils, medium (M)	2 whole
Butternuts	2 to 3
Cashews (M)	4 to 5
Coconut, grated or shredded (S)	2 tablespoons
Filberts or Hazelnuts, whole (M)	5
Hickory, whole, small	5
Macadamia, whole, medium	3
Pecans, chopped (M)	1 tablespoon
Pignolias, whole	1½ tablespoons
Pine Nuts	1 tablespoon
Pistachios (M)	15
Walnuts, chopped (P)	1 tablespoon

SEEDS

Pumpkin Seed Kernels (P)	1 tablespoon
Sesame Seeds (P)	2 teaspoons
Squash Kernels (P)	1 tablespoon
Sunflower Seed Kernels (P)	2 tablespoons

The 1976 revised "Exchange Lists for Meal Planning" divide fats into those which are polyunsaturated and those which are not. The American Heart Association and many other medical groups have been concerned for many years about the undesirably high level of blood lipids (fats) of many Americans. These high levels of lipids are believed to contribute to the development of coronary heart disease. Although there is continuing research, there is general agreement among cardiologists that most of us would be wise to choose more polyunsaturated fats and less saturated ones. They also recommend eating less cholesterol, a fatlike substance found only in animal fats. Because diabetics are statistically even more prone to heart and blood vessel disease than the general population, this dietary modification has been built into the 1976 revision of the Exchanges. Fats are grouped into Polyunsaturated (which tend to lower serum lipids), and Others, a group that includes saturated fats (which tend to raise serum lipids) and monounsaturated fats (which don't change them at all). Clearly the intention is to encourage diabetics to choose polyunsaturated fats instead of saturated fats. To help you plan diets low in saturated fats, all lists are printed with foods high in polyunsaturates and low in saturated fats and cholesterol in boldface type. But there are great individual variations in how your body metabolizes the fats you eat. If your blood lipids are low or normal this might not be important for you. Again, we urge you to talk to your doctor about this. Find out if he feels that a change in your choice of fats is desirable for you on the basis of your own blood lipid values. If so, the information is included in these lists. If not, you don't need to pay any attention as to whether the fats you use are saturated or not.

In the recipe section of this book we have used vegetable oil and margarine instead of butter in all but a few recipes, but you may substitute butter if you wish. This was a decision based on the increasing emphasis on modifying fats. The oil and margarine are also more economical alternatives. Butter and bacon are used only when the product would be more desirable in flavor with their use.

All fats, animal or vegetable, hard or liquid, have nine calories per one gram of pure fat. That means that strictly on a weight basis they are more than twice as fattening as carbohydrates. So be careful to measure your Fat Exchanges or you will have trouble controlling your weight.

Fats, especially margarine, butter, and cream contain Vitamin A in a form that is readily utilized by the body. Vegetable oil is an excellent source of Vitamin E which is needed to prevent destruction of other vitamins and fatty acids. Nuts provide lots of dietary fiber as well as folacin, biotin, zinc and magnesium—all important nutrients needed in very small amounts.

Nondairy Creamers?

You may note that nondairy creamers, powdered or liquid, are not included on the food list. These products are also called coffee whiteners or lighteners. The products differ greatly in food value and many brands are available. Usually 15 grams (½ ounce liquid) provides about 20 calories—surprisingly, more of those calories are from carbohydrate than from fat! The powdered form (1 teaspoon, 2 grams) has 10 to 15 calories including about 1 gram carbohydrate and less than 1 gram of fat. Most of the fat in these products is saturated and monounsaturated. They are *not* recommended for fat-modified diets.

A far better, and less expensive way of "creaming" your coffee is to use 1 teaspoon of instant nonfat dry milk. This is the basis for the most expensive of the prepackaged lighteners and it has almost no fat. In addition to saving lots of money, the instant nonfat dry milk powder needs no refrigeration and has only 10 calories per teaspoon. You may use 1 teaspoon per meal in your beverage without using any Exchanges. If you use more, count 2 teaspoons as ½ of a Fruit Exchange. When using dry milk powder in hot beverages, allow the tea or coffee to cool for a few moments before adding the powder so that the powder will dissolve without a curdled appearance.

7

Free Foods

Another tip for using the Exchange Lists is to remember there are certain foods you can use in unlimited amounts when planning your meals. Some of these include:

Diet Calorie-free Beverage	**Bouillon without fat**
Coffee	**Unsweetened Gelatin**
Tea	**Unsweetened Pickles**

If you like to add seasonings to your food, don't forget there are many you can use freely. Some of the seasonings you may want to consider include:

Salt and Pepper	**Mustard**
Red Pepper	**Chili Powder**
Paprika	**Onion Salt or Powder**
Garlic	**Horseradish**
Celery Salt	**Vinegar**
Parsley	**Mint**
Nutmeg	**Cinnamon**
Lemon	**Lime**

Our Supplementary Free List

These items have only a few calories, less than 20 per serving, and little sugar. They will add variety and flavor to your meals. Some are fine as between-meal snacks. A few of these foods are limited in portion size because larger amounts will use up Exchanges.

BEVERAGES
Beef Tea
Bouillon Cubes, prepared with water
Broth, without fat
Cocoa, dry unsweetened powder (1 tablespoon per day)
Clear consommé
Club Soda, carbonated water
Coffee Lighteners (1 rounded teaspoon per meal)
Decaffeinated Coffee (1 cup per meal)
Fizz Drinks (*see* Index)
Postum (1 rounded teaspoon per meal)
Sauerkraut Juice (½ cup)

SAUCES AND RELISHES
A-1 Sauce or Steak Sauce (1 tablespoon per day)
Catsup, Tomato (1 tablespoon per day)
Chili Sauce (1 tablespoon per day)
Herbed Vinegar
Hot Pepper Sauce
Mustard, prepared (1 tablespoon per day)
Pickles, Dill (1 whole)
Pickles, sour
Pickle Relish, sour or unsweetened
Pimiento (1 tablespoon per day)
Tabasco Sauce
Taco Hot Sauce
Tomato Paste (1 tablespoon per day)
Tomato Puree (1 tablespoon per day)
Worcestershire Sauce
Salad Dressing, Diet (read label and do not exceed 20 calories per
    meal)
Soy Sauce (1 tablespoon per day)

BAKING AIDS
  Baking Powder
  Baking Soda
  Cream of Tartar
  Yeast, Baking
  Pure Flavoring Extracts (Vanilla, Lemon, Almond)

HERBS, SPICES, SEASONINGS
  Achiote Powder
  Allspice
  Basil
  Bay Leaf
  Caraway
  Cayenne Pepper
  Celantro
  Celery Seed, Powder or Juice
  Chili Seeds
  Cloves
  Cumin
  Curry
  Dill
  Ginger
  Ginger Root
  Italian Seasoning
  Marjoram
  Monosodium Glutamate (MSG),
    Accent
  Mustard, Dry
  Onion Juice
  Oregano
  Poppy Seeds
  Poultry Seasoning
  Rosemary
  Sage
  Seasoned Salt
  Tarragon
  Thyme

MISCELLANEOUS
  Gelatin, unflavored plain
  Gelatin Dessert, artificially sweetened (1 cup per day, *see* Index
    for Fruit-Flavored Gel recipes)
  Gum, Sugar-Free
  Jams and Jellies, artificially sweetened (*see* Index for Sweet
    Spreads recipes)
  Lemon Wedge
  Rennet Tablets
  Rhubarb (½ cup, cooked without sugar)
  Yeast, Brewer's (2 teaspoons per day)

8
The Dangerous Dozen

The 1976 revised "Exchange Lists for Meal Planning" states:

The foods in each Exchange List are the familiar, everyday foods you can buy at your supermarket. When you become familiar with the Exchange Lists you will notice that some foods are not mentioned. They have been omitted because they have too much concentrated sugar and may be too high in calories to be safe in your diet. The following foods should not be included in your meal plan without permission of your diet counselor:

Sugar	Syrup
Candy	Condensed Milk
Honey	Chewing Gum
Jam	Soft Drinks
Jelly	Pies
Cookies	Cakes

To that list we also caution you against sweet rolls and coffee cakes. Some bakeries advertise "sugar free" or "dietetic" bakery products but they have often only substituted another sugar, such as honey, for granulated sugar in their recipe. Or they may have added mannitol or sorbitol. These sugars are not encouraged for use by diabetics. Instead use our recipes (*see* Index) for jams, jellies, pies, cakes, and fizz drinks for they are calculated and modified to be safe for you to use. Also "Our Supplementary Bread List" (Chapter 4) contains many commercially available cookies of known nutritive value. See the discussion of the use of these commercial cookies and crackers following that list.

III

Living with Diabetes

9

The Adult with Diabetes

Many factors affect adults with diabetes—the nature and severity of their own diabetes, their family background, education, type of work, and finances. But it is most important for each diabetic not to panic when first diagnosed as having diabetes. Accept the fact, learn about diabetes, talk about it, ask your doctor and diet counselor all kinds of questions, and read when and what you can. Because the foods you eat and your meal plans are truly the foundation of successful diabetes management, we urge you to learn more and more about foods for the diabetic. There are many people and places willing and able to help you. But, actually, it all boils down to *you*. Your doctor and your diet counselor will tell you that you are basically responsible for yourself. They can give you all the information you need but you make all the decisions in your day-to-day care.

Parents and other family members and friends can be very helpful. Their understanding and patience can encourage you. But don't let anyone coax you into breaking the rules. Don't hide the fact that you are now a diabetic. Stand up to it, talk about it, and you'll be very surprised at the warm understanding that will surround you. As you become increasingly aware of your diabetes and its successful management, you will gain confidence, enjoy a wide selection of foods (such as our recipes), and perhaps be a greater achiever than you have ever been before!

51

10

The Child with Diabetes

On "Sesame Street," Kermit the Frog sings a song "It's Not Easy Being Green." That song tells a story of how difficult it is to be different. The child who has diabetes is different from other children and it's not easy—for either the child or for his parents.

Almost every child at some point feels different, unacceptable to others and to himself. Sometimes it's because he's too fat, too skinny, has acne, wears glasses, has asthma, or walks with a limp. Children who have diabetes have a medical problem that is not easily cured by modern medicine. So far, the answer is control—by both insulin and diet.

In the very young child, the responsibility lies mostly with the parents. Many parents feel guilty because of the hereditary aspect of diabetes and they become overly protective. Children, whether diabetic or not, quickly learn that they can manipulate parents by eating or not eating, by eating the right foods or the wrong ones, or by behaving or misbehaving to get attention. Very often the child thinks that he or she is the only child in the whole world with diabetes.

Summer Camps

To help overcome this feeling of being different is one of the many values of a summer camp for diabetic children. There are over 50 summer camps for children with diabetes in the United States. Most of them include all of the normal camping activities such as swimming, boating, horseback riding, games, and physical exercises under instruction and supervision. But they also are staffed with complete health teams, doctors, dietitians, and nurses who supervise, teach, and help every child. The camps often have junior counselors who may or may not be diabetics or who may have a family interest in diabetes. One of the greatest experiences for the child is the meeting with other diabetic children, talking together, learning together, and finding out that they are not alone with their problems. Although there has to be a not-for-profit charge for each child, usually no child's application is refused because the parents cannot pay. The camp committee's main consideration is which of the applicants needs camp the most. Write to the American Diabetes Association, Inc. (see address under Sources of Information), and ask for a list of Summer Camps for Diabetic Children, in or near your state.

In addition to the physical benefits of summer camp, it is often a good idea to get the child away from the parents for a few weeks. During this separation the child can experience a great deal of personal growth and can develop independent behavior and self-confidence in a safe environment. Also the parents may get a much-needed rest or vacation with other family members who may not have been getting their fair share of attention.

The Parents' Role

It helps, in the long run, to encourage the child to assume as much responsibility as possible for his or her own care. The doctor or nurse will help teach the child how to give his own insulin at the appropriate time.

Often the parents, especially the mother, are particularly involved in the management of the diet. Even young children can be taught the basic Exchanges. It is much like many board games that they play. The child can help prepare meals, weigh and cut his food portions, pack lunches and so on. The diet counselor will work with the child and his parents. An ongoing relationship with a diet counselor is important.

You can teach the child that his diabetes is a fact not a secret. Share the fact with others who will be supportive. Let the parents of his playmates know that the child has diabetes and send appropriate food and snacks if necessary. Be sure that others don't misinterpret "I'm not allowed to have candy at home," to mean that the child deserves more treats when he comes over to play.

As the child gets older, more self-directed, and more accepting of his diabetes, there will be continued peaks and valleys. The adolescent, whether diabetic or not, will seek limits, defy authority, and test new behavior. Hormonal changes cause spurts of growth which change insulin and food needs. The diabetes may seem to be less in control. Often discussion groups, much like those held at summer camp, will be useful for kids with diabetes as well as other long-term medical problems.

Some parents have been able to create an emotional environment that makes their child, who happens to be diabetic, feel special rather than sick or odd. The emotional and physical needs of just being a child are far more important than those of being a diabetic. But don't forget Kermit who said "It's not easy . . . . "

11
Exercise and Sports

You may wonder why we have included this section in a book about the dietary control of diabetes. Well, calories come in through diet but they need a bit of help from physical activity to get out.

From a simply caloric standpoint, all of us, whether we are diabetic or not, maintain our weight from the calories we eat as balanced by the energy it takes to run our sophisticated motor of a body plus our physical activity. In other words, we can eat more (without gaining weight) if we are physically active. On the other hand, we must eat less if we get little physical exercise. Maintaining a desirable or ideal weight is important to diabetics. Lean bodies use insulin more effectively and, if insulin is necessary, less is needed at ideal weight.

The insulin-dependent diabetic must remember that exercise causes the muscles to use blood sugar independent of insulin action. So the insulin-dependent diabetic must either reduce his insulin dosage or consume some sugar prior to vigorous exercise. This is one of the rare times that sweetened pop, candy, honey, or fruit juice between meals can be taken. Also, the insulin-dependent diabetic should carry with him additional sources of sugar in case more sugar is needed in the middle of the activity. The physician will plan appropriate sugar sources with you.

Many great athletes have been and are insulin-dependent diabetics. Children with diabetes should be encouraged to participate in active sports as well as other school programs. Certainly the gym teacher, classroom teacher, school nurse, lunchroom personnel, and school bus drivers should be informed that a student has diabetes. Parents are wise to provide them with a list of symptoms of hypoglycemia and ask them to be especially watchful just before lunchtime. Make sure that strenuous physical activity is not scheduled immediately before lunchtime. Before strenuous activity, such as football practice or tennis, be sure that the child takes extra sugar or that he has taken less insulin. Send some packets of sugar to the teacher to keep available.

Full participation in sports and school activities is very important to all children, whether they happen to have diabetes or not. The child with diabetes can do everything a nondiabetic child can—with planning and care and encouragement.

12
Eating Out

People like to eat out sometimes. In fact, the National Restaurant Association estimates that one out of every three meals in the United States is eaten away from home, and they predict this trend to continue. Fast food restaurants are found everywhere. Many workers have to eat out every workday if it is not possible for them to carry lunch with them. For the diabetic who has done his homework, that is, learned what he can eat and how much, choosing from menus is not too difficult. Even if someone else cooks for you at home, as a diabetic you should know the foods and portion sizes on your diabetic diet.

Kay says one must have a few ground rules, and here are hers:

- Don't be tempted by the gorgeous goodies you are used to choosing from menus unless you have the will power to eat very small portions and you include the estimated values in your meal.
- Make up your own pocket- or purse-sized cards of the Food Exchange lists. These cards will help you to select from menus.
- Just because the restaurant chef serves large portions doesn't mean you must clean the plate. Eat only the amount your diabetic diet

will allow—share with someone, leave the rest, or ask for a doggie bag to take home for another meal.
- Tell the waitress that you are a diabetic and ask her to tell the chef to "go easy on the fats."

And now, to guide you along the menu route from beginning to end:

APPETIZERS.   Skip all cream soups, creamed herring, etc. If you choose seafood (shrimp) cocktail count it as part of your total meal's Meat Exchange. A few celery sticks, a radish, or a carrot curl from a relish tray could be considered "free." Clear beef or chicken soup is fine. Tomato juice, vegetable juice, or vegetable soup are allowed only if you count a Vegetable Exchange. Or use a Fruit Exchange for a small fresh fruit cup or melon wedge.

BREADS.   Limit your choice to one small, plain roll, ½ large roll, melba toast, or breadsticks. Count them for an allowed Bread Exchange. Breads add up fast, so be sure to count them! If you use butter or margarine, count Fat Exchanges.

SALADS AND DRESSING.   Choose a green salad garnished with a wedge of lemon or sliced tomato and count it as a Vegetable Exchange. If you have extra fat allowance remember that 1 tablespoon French or Italian dressing is worth 1 Fat Exchange. If you are a regular patron of a certain restaurant, ask them to keep a jar of your favorite homemade dressing for you. Mark it with your name and give it to the waitress to refrigerate. After all, they save partial bottles of wine for customers in France!

MAIN COURSE FOR LUNCH.   Depending upon your bread allowance, consider an open-face sandwich (1 slice), a regular sandwich (2 slices), or a club sandwich (3 slices). The best fillings are lean meat, sliced chicken or turkey, or cheese. Avoid fried sandwiches. Other main lunch choices could include: cottage cheese, deviled eggs, sliced cheese, strips of meat and cheese on a green salad, or a broiled beef patty; however, no gravies, sauces, cream cheese fillings, or salad fillings with lots of mayonnaise as a binder.

MAIN COURSE FOR DINNER. Choose lean meat, fish, or poultry—roasted, baked, grilled, broiled, or poached. Trim off extra fats from chops, steaks, and sliced meats. Avoid thickened gravies and cream sauces.

VEGETABLES. Keep in mind the Vegetable Exchange list (½ cup). Ask if they have a fresh vegetable of the day. Avoid cream sauces, cheese sauces, and fried vegetables. Did you already use the allowed vegetables in your salad or appetizers?

POTATOES. Got your pocket or purse list handy? Check to see what kind of potato dishes you may have and how much. Consider rice or pasta alternatives as Bread Exchanges. Skip French fries, potato chips, and butter or sour cream on potatoes, unless you have lots of Fat Exchanges to use.

DESSERTS. Fresh fruit is by far the best choice. But if you have been very, very, good and your doctor permits you to have plain ice cream once in a while, ask for 1 very small (½ cup) scoop of plain vanilla, coffee, strawberry, or chocolate ice cream and count it as 1 Bread Exchange plus 2 Fat Exchanges. Restaurant cakes, pies, pastries, custards, puddings, sherbets, water ices are definitely not for diabetics. They have far too much sugar!

Good eating!

13

Alcohol for Diabetics?

Adult diabetics frequently ask whether they can have a drink before dinner. There is no standard answer to this. So much depends upon the severity of the diabetes condition, the individual, and the physician's knowledge as to whether the diabetic fully understands (1) what the permissive "occasionally" means, (2) that whatever alcoholic beverage is taken is counted in along with the food, and (3) that other sources of calories must be omitted at the same meal.

It just makes good sense that, because your calories are restricted, every calorie should carry nutrients for good health. Also, for the diabetic whose medication is insulin, and whose meal schedule must be regular, there is a real danger. The relaxing effect of a before-dinner drink just might relax you right past your regular mealtime, and put you in danger of an insulin reaction. Or you may eat far too much or the wrong foods after a drink or two.

Consult your own physician as to whether you may have an occasional drink. Find out whether he considers hard liquor or wine to be suitable. The following material is reprinted from "A Guide for Professionals" prepared by Committees of the American Diabetes Association, Inc., and the American Dietetic Association and is used with their permission.

Alcohol

Alcohol is quickly absorbed and contributes seven calories per gram. Although it is not converted into sugar or acetone, its caloric content may be responsible for gain in weight. It may cause hypoglycemia in the patient with insulin-dependent diabetes, especially if meals are missed or delayed. Therefore, the consumption of alcohol should be discussed with the patient's physician.

Considerations in the Use of Alcoholic Beverages

A. Use alcohol only when the diabetes is under control.
B. Because alcohol has blood sugar lowering ability under some circumstances, use alcohol only with meals and snacks, and in moderation *only*.
C. Avoid sweet wines, liqueurs, beer, ale, and sweetened mixed drinks because of their high sugar content.
D. Avoid alcohol if on a weight reduction diet, because alcohol provides calories and stimulates the appetite.

Exchanges for Alcoholic Beverages

Because alcohol is metabolized to two-carbon fragments and handled by the body as fat, it may be calculated as a substitute for an appropriate number of Fat Exchanges. One Fat Exchange should be removed for every 45 calories contained in the alcoholic beverage being used. However, if an individual is at ideal body weight, he may wish to use alcohol as extra calories without subtracting Fat Exchanges. The following formula can be applied to calculate the number of calories: $0.8 \times \text{proof} \times \text{ounces} = \text{calories}$.

Liquor: gin, rum, scotch,
   vodka, whiskey   1½ oz. = 2 to 3 Fat Exchanges (80 proof = 96 calories; 100 proof = 120 calories)
Dry Wine
   (unsweetened)   3½ oz. = 1½ Fat Exchanges (approx. 70 calories)
Beer (low-caloric)   12 oz. = 2 Fat Exchanges (approx. 90 calories)

Wines in Cooking?

You will see that some of our recipes use wine as an ingredient. In each case the carbohydrate values have been calculated into the total for the recipe. Where the recipe is cooked, and the calories from the alcohol in the wine have been cooked away, only the calories from the carbohydrates and the carbohydrates themselves are included in the total nutritive values. In those few "no-cook" recipes using wine, the total calorie values of the wines, both from carbohydrate and alcohol, are included.

14

Food Exchanges for Fast Foods*

Arthur Treacher's

2-piece fish dinner (fish, chips, coleslaw)
3 High-Fat Meats, plus 4 Breads, plus 1 Vegetable, plus 2 Fruits, plus 5 Fats, total of 905 calories.**

Long John Silver's

2-piece fish dinner (fish, chips, coleslaw)
3½ High-Fat Meats, plus 4½ Breads, plus 2½ Vegetables, plus 4 Fats, plus 1 Fruit, total of 944 calories.**

Burger Chef

Hamburger
1½ High-Fat Meats, plus 1 Bread, plus 1 Fruit, total of 258 calories.

Big Shef
3 High-Fat Meats, plus 3 Breads, plus 1 Fat, total of 549 calories.

French Fries
2 Breads, plus 2½ Fats, total of 249 calories.

Chocolate Shake
½ Milk, plus 2 Fats, plus 1 Fruit, plus 2 Breads, total of 306 calories.

Burger King

Hamburger — 2 Medium-Fat Meats, plus 1 Bread, plus 1 Fruit, total 243 calories.

Whopper — 3 High-Fat Meats, plus 3 Breads, plus 2 Fats, plus ½ Fruit, total 614 calories.

French Fries — 2 Breads, plus 2 Fats, total 226 calories.

Chocolate Shake — 4 Breads, plus ½ Fruit, plus 1½ Fats, total 360 calories.

McDonald's

Hamburger — 1½ Medium-Fat Meats, plus 2 Breads, total 252 calories.

Big Mac — 2 High-Fat Meats, plus 2½ Breads, plus 1 Vegetable, plus 3 Fats, total of 533 calories.

French Fries — 1 Bread, plus 1 Vegetable, plus 2 Fats, total of 186 calories.

Chocolate Shake — 1 Milk, plus 2 Fats, plus 2 Breads, plus 1 Fruit, total of 346 calories.

Kentucky Fried Chicken

2-piece original — 4 Lean Meats, plus 3 Breads, plus 3 Fats, plus 1 Vegetable, total of 587 calories.

2-piece crispy — 4 Medium-Fat Meats, plus 2½ Breads, plus 1 Vegetable, plus 3 Fats, total of 643 calories

Pizza Hut

Individuals
Thick Crust — 8 Breads, plus 1 Milk, plus 2 Vegetables, plus 6 Lean Meats, total of 1026 calories.**

Thin Crust — 8 Breads, plus 2 Vegetables, plus 6 Lean Meats, plus 2 Fats, total of 1020 calories.**

* Food Exchanges calculated from nutrient data in the May-June 1976 "Diabetes Forecast."

** Few diabetics have this many Exchanges to use at one meal. How about sharing and reducing calories and Exchange Values in half?

15
Traveling?

By all means. Don't stay at home just because you are a diabetic. Many insulin-dependent diabetics, young and older, have tripped and traveled all over the world. Professional sportsmen such as Bobby Clarke (hockey), Ron Santo (baseball), Mike Pyle (football), and Bill Talbert (tennis) have successfully dealt with their insulin-dependent diabetes while playing vigorously and traveling endlessly. One of our favorite stars, Mary Tyler Moore never has allowed her diabetes condition to stop her dancing, acting, and traveling. "If they can do it, why not you and me," says Kay! Here are a few reminders:

- In your purse or pocket carry a letter from your physician stating your diabetes condition, your medication, and your doctor's name, address, and telephone number including area code. If you take insulin, the letter should explain to the border customs agent why you have syringes and needles. In this age of drugs, they are suspicious, especially of the young.
- Wear an identification bracelet or insignia on a neck chain to indicate that you have diabetes. These are worldwide signals to

medical personnel. Mary's cousin was a juvenile diabetic who refused to wear identification and several times she had emergencies and was thought to be drunk! But this was entirely avoidable.

- From your state or local affiliate of the American Diabetes Association, Inc., get several diabetes identification wallet cards. Fill them out, put one in purse or pocket, another in a suitcase, and give another to a friend who is traveling with you. Ask them also for any pamphlets they may have about traveling tips.
- Carry your insulin or other medications with you. Luggage can be separated from you or even lost. What you carry on your person is always with you.
- If the timing of your meals is strictly regulated and you expect to travel to areas in a different time zone, talk to your doctor or diet counselor for help in making your mealtime adjustments.
- When making air travel reservations it is important to tell your travel agent or reservation clerk that you are a diabetic and will require diabetic menus on flights. (Kay says that other passengers are envious of her attractive diabetic meals, they are that delicious!)
- Take copies of your meal plans and Food Exchange Lists with you. Also be guided by our suggestions in "Eating Out" (Chapter 12).
- Carry with you for emergencies a roll of Lifesavers or other hard candy. They are easier to carry than sugar cubes. Don't forget that sweetened pop is sold all over the world, and is permitted for certain diabetic emergencies.
- When you stay in a foreign country, register at the American Embassy or Consular Office; they can assist you to get medical help if you need it. Also, your doctor can provide you with a list of physicians in each country who assist foreign travelers, speak English, and charge standard fees.

Happy Holiday!

16

Shopping for Food

With today's food prices, most of us need to be concerned about food costs in relation to the family's food needs. Since there is a diabetic in the family, this person's needs are especially important. However, if we remember that a well-planned diet for the diabetic provides all nutrients, it can be the basis for good nutrition for the whole family.

Wise food shopping is a part of the art of good cooking. And, because the recipes in this book are entirely suitable and delicious for the whole family, why not let the diabetic's menus be a guide for planning the family menus? Make whatever adjustments for the rest of the family you may think necessary.

Before You Shop

• Plan the diabetic's menus for several days in advance. Make a grocery list and add whatever additional items you want for the family, always considering the *must* items first.

- Keep the list flexible so that you may take advantage of any unadvertised suitable foods at bargain prices. For example, a sudden markdown on juice oranges might make them a better buy than the juice itself.
- Make your list from your menus, grouping the foods together that you will find in the same areas of the store. This saves needless running around the store. Kay writes her list on the backs of old envelopes that hold clipped coupons.

When You Shop

- If possible, do your food shopping soon after a meal. Studies show we spend ⅓ more when we shop when hungry. Temptations jump into the market basket!
- Buy first what you really need; avoid impulse buying. The first concern should be for the foods for the diabetic and good nutrition for the family. If money is left, then add less nutritious snacks and treats.
- Read labels very carefully; and that brings us to the next chapter, "How to Read a Label."

17

How to Read a Label

For years, consumers have been demanding more and more information about the nutritive values of the foods we eat. In answer to these demands the Food and Drug Administration, in 1973, developed a standardized form for nutritional labeling. At present, this program is voluntary, which means that unless the food processor adds nutrients to the product or makes dietary claims on the label, he is not required to provide nutrition information on the package. As expected, many of the most nutritious foods provide labels that indicate this while producers of foods with very little nutrient value except for calories are less likely to provide the consumer with full information.

Nutritional labeling is an important tool to diabetics and others on special diets. It is very useful to know the carbohydrate, protein, fat, and calorie levels of foods that we buy so that processed foods can be translated into Exchanges and fit into the diet.

If a product does not have a nutritional label you can write to the packer and ask for nutrition information. Many companies (Campbell Soups, Heinz Products, Kellogg, General Mills, Beatrice Foods, and others) will be happy to send you the nutritive content of their products. Some companies, such as Campbell Soups, even have their product information translated into Diabetic Food Exchanges for you.

But how do we interpret nutritional labeling when it is provided? First, let's look at a label for V-8 Cocktail Vegetable Juice:

NUTRITION INFORMATION
PER SERVING

Serving Size..6 oz.
Servings Per Container...2
Calories...35
Protein...1 Gram
Carbohydrate ....7 Grams
Fat...0 Grams

PERCENT OF U.S. RECOMMENDED
DAILY ALLOWANCE (U.S. RDA)

Protein	2	Riboflavin	2
Vitamin A	35	Niacin	6
Vitamin C	45	Calcium	2
Thiamine	4	Iron	2

NET 12 FL. OZ. (354 ml.)

INGREDIENTS:

Tomato juice or reconstituted tomato juice, plus juices of carrots, celery, beets, parsley, lettuce, watercress, spinach, with salt, ascorbic acid (Vitamin C) and natural flavoring.

Campbell Soup Company,
Camden, N.J. U.S.A. 08101

Note that the first section of the label tells the serving size, the number of servings in the container, the calories per serving, and the grams of carbohydrate, protein, and fat per serving. This information can then be evaluated to determine into which Food Exchange List the product fits. Sometimes, the identified standard serving size suggested by the packer does not fit into an even amount for an Exchange. We know from List 2—Vegetable Exchanges that a ½-cup serving, 4 ounces, would be one Vegetable Exchange. So the diabetic would get 3 Vegetable Exchanges, 4 ounces each, from the 12-ounce can instead of the suggested 2 servings at 6 ounces. The 4-ounce serving would yield 5 grams of carbohydrate, 1 gram protein, 0 Fat, and 25 calories. Perfect!

The packer determines the standard portion size for each product. Sometimes far too generous servings are suggested by the packers. Other times tiny servings are set so the packer can claim very small caloric values per serving. We found a label on a 4½-ounce box of "dietetic imitation chocolate covered raisins" that claimed very low caloric and carbohydrate values. Then we discovered the reason for these values. The packer claimed that there were 20 servings in the box. We wonder how many diabetics and weightwatchers ate a whole box of that "dietetic" candy! This product, in which the only modification was to substitute imitation chocolate for real chocolate, had even more calories and fat than the product that it was supposed to replace. Its only real use would be if there was an allergy or intolerance to chocolate. But the product was very deceiving as well as expensive.

The next section of the label lists percentages of the U.S. Recommended Daily Allowances (U.S. RDA). This part of nutrition labeling is more difficult to understand. The U.S. RDA's are our goals for good nutrition. If you eat 100% of the identified nutrient from all foods in a given day you will more than meet your need for that nutrient. The percentages indicate, on the vegetable juice cocktail label, that this product is a very good source of Vitamin C and Vitamin A and provides small amounts of other vitamins and minerals. But the 2, 4 and 6 percents do add up to contribute to your daily need.

The third section of the label is the ingredient list. The law requires that ingredients always be listed in order of weight. So, because it's listed first, you know that there is more tomato juice than any other single ingredient in the can. You also learn that there is more carrot juice than celery juice because of the order in which they appear on the ingredient list.

Even products without complete nutritional labeling are required by law to provide a complete list of ingredients in order of weight. Always check the ingredient list for sources of sugar. See "The Great Sugar Masquerade" (Chapter 19) for the list of sugars you should be careful to avoid. The ingredients list also will include any nutrient additions or chemicals added to the food. Sometimes the specific type of fat is identified, corn oil for example, or the more general term vegetable oil may be used. If you are on a fat-modified diet look for sources of polyunsaturated fats.

The last required item on nutritional labeling is the packer or processor's name and address.

There are several other things that a label may include, but these are optional. Milligrams of sodium, cholesterol, or type of fat may be included. If a claim is made that a product is low in sodium, the level of sodium must be listed.

Some foods are labeled "dietetic." This only means that they are somehow altered. You must then carefully read the label. Maybe the vegetable is packed without salt. But the words "dietetic" or "calorie controlled" or "sugar restricted" do not mean that the diabetic can eat unlimited quantities of that food! Remember those raisins?

On the labels of some "dietetic" foods the nutritive values are marked by a system based on % by volume. This is confusing to many diabetics who think that, for example, the 20% of carbohydrate labeled equals 20 grams of carbohydrate. If there are products labeled in % by volume that you want to use, ask your diet counselor to translate the values into grams of carbohydrate, protein, and fat, and into Exchanges.

18

Brown Bag Foods

Frequently, it's easier for a diabetic child or adult to carry lunch in a brown bag than to choose food in a school cafeteria or restaurant. At home you have both the food and the time to make sure that the correct Food Exchanges are included. "Brown Baggers," as we sometimes call today's lunch carriers, do get tired of the roast beef sandwich and canned-soup routine! And who blames them!

As with any meal, look at the meal plan and choose the combination of foods to equal your allowed number of Food Exchanges. If you are choosing a stew with 2 Meat Exchanges and 1 Bread Exchange and you are allowed 3 Meat Exchanges and 2 Bread Exchanges, then fill in with a piece of bread and 1 ounce of cheese. Check the lunch to make sure that you have used all of your allotted Exchanges.

One of the big problems, of course, is where can the lunch be stored at school or work? Sometimes a refrigerator is available. If not, be sure that there is no mayonnaise filling that could spoil. If the diabetic lunch-carrier is willing to carry a wide-mouth thermos and a 1-cup beverage thermos, the problem is more than half solved.

There are many recipes in this book which may be packed into the wide-mouth thermos and be hot for lunch. To find the recipes, look in the Index.

Beef Porcupines in Tomato Gravy	Old-Fashioned Beef Stew
Chicken a la King	Fish Chowder
Chicken Chow Mein	Cream of Tomato Soup
Chili Con Carne	Mushroom Vegetable Soup
Sloppy Joes	Hearty Vegetable Soup
Lamb Curry	Chicken Giblet and Vegetable Soup

Or, you may pack chicken, sliced meat loaf, cold meats, or cheese directly in foil. If you choose one of the meat dishes, to the carried lunch add some celery and carrot sticks wrapped in plastic wrap. If you select one of the hearty soups, add a protein-type sandwich or cheese and a roll. As to sandwiches, some of our breads and sandwich fillings (*see* Index) are delicious for brown bag or picnic lunches.

Milk Exchanges tend to cause problems because they require refrigeration or a thermos. Children can buy milk at most schools. That saves carrying it and the problem of keeping it chilled. Adults often use their Milk Exchanges at other times during the day. V-8, tomato juice, fruit juice, coffee, or tea may be alternate beverages. If there is a Milk Exchange available, Hot Milk Chocolate (*see* Index) will be a favorite beverage in cold weather.

Don't forget to include raw vegetables to nibble or cooked ones put in the thermos. Salads or mixed raw vegetables may be packed in a plastic bag or in a 10-ounce paper cup. Envelopes of single servings of dressing are also sold in some markets so look for them.

Look at List 3—Fruit Exchanges. Pack the appropriate amount of any fresh fruit in season. Fresh or dried fruits pack far better than frozen or canned ones, which can easily leak. Look in your market for individual cans of unsweetened juices if you want to use a Fruit Exchange as your beverage.

If the diabetic member of your family requires midmorning and/or midafternoon snacks, and there is no good source at school or work where the suitable snacks may be purchased, then these must be a part of the packed lunch. For a child, ask the teacher to keep the crackers or appropriate snack at school. Often the child can bring 5 small bags, a snack for each day, at the beginning of the week and keep it somewhere at school. The child can then be excused daily to go eat his snack. This is often better for both the child and classmates than eating it in the classroom.

19

The Great Sugar Masquerade

The word "sugar" to most people means only white table sugar or brown sugar. But there are really over 100 sweet substances which can be described as sugars. All of these sweet substances are carbohydrates—an enormous family of nutrients that provide most of the energy in our diet. Carbohydrates come in four forms:

Sugars: The smallest and sweetest members of the carbohydrate family. They are found in all sweets and in fruits.
Starches: Chemically these are long chains of sugars that are usually not sweet. They are found in grains, cereal, potatoes, pasta products, and baked goods. After digestion they are broken down into sugars for use in the human body.
Indigestible Carbohydrates: Cellulose and others which give fiber and bulk. Our body does not have the enzyme to break this down so no sugar is released when we eat cellulose.
Sugar Alcohols: Synthetic products made from sugars or cellulose, and, although the digestive system metabolizes these slower than it does sugar, these products end up in the body as sugar. The most popular ones are sorbitol, mannitol, and xylitol.

Although diabetics are cautioned about the use of carbohydrates, we learn that everyone, even those with the most serious and difficult to control diabetes, must have some carbohydrates every day, because this food family is such an important source of quick energy and our brain and nervous system require carbohydrates as their fuel

100 Sugars?

What about all those 100 sweet substances? Well, we don't need to know all their names, but there are several that every diabetic should know about, just to be able to recognize the hidden sugars on lists of ingredients on labels. One of the quick tricks is to look for "ose" words, because this helps tell you of the presence of a sugar. Like these:

Sucrose: Sometimes called saccharose. There is white sugar (cane or beet sugar), granulated, cubed, or powdered, that gives us nothing but calories; brown sugar, much less refined, derived from molasses (sorghum cane), that gives us very small amounts of a few minerals; and raw sugar, very similar to brown sugar, sometimes crystalline. There is also a new product called "liquid brown sugar."

Fructose: Sometimes called levulose. It is found in free form in fruits and in honey. It is highly soluble and very much sweeter than any other sugar in equal amounts. You may also see on a label "High Fructose Syrup," which is a concentrated form of fructose.

Lactose: Sometimes called milk sugar because milk is its chief food source. It is a combination of glucose and galactose.

Galactose: This is a simple sugar found in lactose.

Dextrose: Commercially obtained from starch; sometimes called corn sugar or grape sugar.

Glucose: Found chiefly in fruits, some vegetables, honey, and corn syrup. Starches break down to glucose, and all other sugars convert to glucose, the form of carbohydrate that the body uses. The phrase "blood glucose" refers to the level of sugar in the blood.

Maltose: Comes from the breakdown of starch in the malting of barley. When starches are digested they pass through a stage of being maltose before they end up as glucose.

Mannose: Comes from manna and the ivory nut; used mostly by sugar chemists. Mannitol is derived from mannose.

Although these "ose" sugars have different names, because of their sweet flavor they are used to sweeten foods. And, we must never forget that, whether we use them alone or with other ingredients, each of these "ose" sugars is a carbohydrate; and every 1 gram gives us 4 calories. Concentrated sources of sugar must be limited by the diabetic.

Other Familiar Sugars

Besides the names given in the "ose" group there are other names we need to recognize as being sugars.

Corn Syrup: A liquid form of corn sugar, it is used in baking and infant feeding formulas; when crystallized it may be called corn syrup solids or corn sweetener. It is relatively inexpensive and is used to make syrup for canned fruits.
Maple Syrup: And maple sugar; made from the sap of maple trees.
Molasses: And sorghum; made from sorghum canes.
Honey: Comes from floral sources from which bees collect nectar; it comes liquid, creamed, and in combs; it is a more concentrated form of carbohydrates than table sugars. Some health food stores and magazines have told diabetics that they may eat honey instead of sugar because it does not require insulin to be metabolized. This is not true because the honey is converted to glucose like all other sugars and insulin is then needed. Don't be fooled! Honey must be considered a carbohydrate.

Sugar Alcohols?

The sugar alcohols have had to be adopted into the sugar family because, although they are chemically alcohols, they are commercially made from some of the "ose" sugars. Any used for human consumption are much more slowly digested and absorbed than are sugars, but they do end up in the body as carbohydrates and therefore must be counted into the diabetic diet.

You will see these names among ingredients:

Sorbitol: Commercially made from glucose; used widely in the commercial manufacture of dietetic foods and sugar-free gum.
Mannitol and **Dulcitol:** Manufactured from mannose and galactose.
Xylitol: Manufactured from xylose (wood sugar), found in corn cobs, straw, bran, woodgum, and the bran of seeds. Xylose has been identified in fruits such as cherries, pears, peaches, and plums. As with the other sugar alcohols, xylitol is slowly absorbed, but the amount absorbed by the body contributes calories. Some chewing gums contain xylitol because it is not supposed to cause tooth decay. This is still being studied.

There is some caution suggested in eating foods sweetened with sorbitol, mannitol, and xylitol, however. Many people, upon eating generous amounts of sugar alcohols, develop gastrointestinal problems such as diarrhea. In a diabetic this can be especially serious.

Fructose As an Alternative Sweetener

Fructose, as mentioned earlier, is a natural sugar found in fruits and honey. When sucrose breaks down in our body, it yields glucose and fructose.

In Europe, especially in West Germany and Switzerland, pure fructose is accepted as a sweetener for use by diabetics. There, it is called "non-glucose carbohydrate." Many foods are now being introduced to our markets which contain fructose, so you should understand what fructose does, and its advantages and limitations for use by diabetics.

Fructose is absorbed more slowly than glucose into the bloodstream. It does raise the level of sugar in the blood, but not as quickly, nor to the same level, as equal amounts of glucose. Unlike glucose, most fructose is metabolized in the liver. This means that it does not require an initial insulin response to get it from the blood directly into the cells for metabolism. During metabolism, part of the molecule may be formed into glucose. At this point, some insulin is required. But the entire process of fructose absorption and metabolism requires far less insulin than the use of equal amounts of glucose.

While this sounds good for diabetics, it must be remembered that fructose is still a carbohydrate and must always be carefully used, because it has the same caloric value as other sugars. The use of limited amounts of foods containing fructose seems to be safe. However, excessive use, or the use of fructose cake frostings and similar sweets, is most unwise unless you are one of the rare diabetics with an exceptionally high caloric need.

Some medical research suggests that fructose consumption may increase uric acid production, and this is a potential problem for those with gout. There is very limited research data at present regarding the long-term effect of high levels of fructose in the diets of diabetics.

Because the use of fructose is still controversial, do consult your doctor or diet counselor before adding fructose to your diet. For more information on added fructose, see page 82.

20
Sugar Substitutes

At the time this book goes to press, the battle over saccharin is not over. We are confident that even if the Food and Drug Administration bans saccharin from use by the general public, it will still be available for use by diabetics. And if a full ban goes into effect, it won't happen until an alternative artificial sweetener is available. Because the availability of diet pops, artificially sweetened gelatin products, and artificially sweetened jams and jellies is in question, we have included recipes (*see* Index for Fruit-Flavored Gels and Sweet Spreads) for many of these products. We think that once you try them you will find them far more delicious than the commercial products now available.

At this time there are two types of artificially sweetened products to choose from: "No Calorie" sugar substitutes are entirely saccharin-based with no additional sweetening agent. They have no nutritive values of any kind. Many saccharin products contain sodium. If a Low-Sodium Diet is prescribed, choose an artificial sweetener that does not contain sodium. Many other preparations are called "Lo Calorie," because they contain lactose, dextrose, or some other carbohydrates or sugar alcohols (mannitol, sorbitol, or xylitol.) All of these have some carbohydrate and calorie values. Even in small amounts, they should be considered by the diabetic and built in to his calculated diet. Reading labels is particularly important with these products.

You will note that many of our recipes call for "artificial sweetener to substitute for ___ amount of sugar." How much is that? It depends upon the brand you use and its concentration of sweetening power. So, our two tips are:

• Read the label of your artificial sweetener carefully because it will tell you how much of that particular artificial sweetener will serve in place of how much sugar.
• Read the label carefully to find out if your artificial sweetener contains any of the "ose" sugars listed in "The Great Sugar Masquerade" (Chapter 19), and if so, the label must tell you how many grams carbohydrates and how many calories yielded by ___ amount of that artificial sweetener. Multiply the amounts given by how much you need to use in the recipe; then add those total grams carbohydrates and total calories to the carbohydrate and calories provided by the other ingredients to calculate your serving.

Some of the sugar substitutes presently on the market tell you:

GRANULAR FORM. 1 envelope equals 1 teaspoon of sugar in sweetness; or 1 envelope equals 2 teaspoons of sugar in sweetness; or 1 teaspoon equals 1 teaspoon of sugar in sweetness.

TABLET FORM. 1 tablet (¼ grain size) equals 1 teaspoon of sugar in sweetness.

LIQUID FORM. ⅛ teaspoon equals 1 teaspoon of sugar in sweetness; or 2 drops equals 1 teaspoon of sugar in sweetness.

These are only examples, based on some of the brands we have used. As new sugar substitutes come on the market read the labels carefully to know how much to use. Perhaps your diet counselor will help you make a chart to put in this book which will tell you the following:

For Amount Sugar	*Your Favorite Sugar Substitute*
1 teaspoon	1 tablet
3 teaspoons (1 tablespoon)	3 tablets
¼ cup	12 tablets
⅓ cup	16 tablets
½ cup	24 tablets

Then, when you need this information for any of our recipes you will have it handy. If you use tablet forms, crush them thoroughly. Most sugar substitutes are better added after a food is heated or cooked. If added during the cooking period the chemicals can break down to develop a bitter rather than sweet taste. That's why our recipes usually add the artificial sweetener at the very end of the directions.

Fructose

Fructose, while a naturally occurring sugar, is being used as an alternative to artificial sweeteners in the production of many foods for special diets. Batter-Lite Foods, Inc. has developed several cakes, cookies, frosting mixes, and spreads, and you may have seen these products (or those made by other manufacturers) in stores or advertized in *Diabetes Forecast*. For diabetics, fructose is a "mixed blessing." Again, we remind you to check with your doctor or diet counselor before deciding if you should use foods with added fructose. As indicated on page 79, you may want to ask which of these foods you may use, how often, and the appropriate portion size. Foods with added fructose are never "Free Foods," they must be substituted for other foods in your meal plan.

When using pure fructose as a sugar substitute, keep in mind that it is a carbohydrate. Read the label on the box or individual packet to find out the carbohydrate and calorie level in the amount you may wish to use. Because fructose is somewhat sweeter than other sugars, less may be required for the same sweet flavor.

21

Sugar in Our Recipes?

Almost all of our recipes that need something to give the finished product a sweet flavor include a sugar substitute. Often, they also call for a larger-than-usual measure of vanilla, which does add flavor too. But, neither of these "tricks" will work in baked products which need a real sugar not only for flavor and tenderness but also for proper browning. It is a well-known fact that the regular sugar used in making cakes and cookies is required not only for sweet taste but also for its chemical action in combination with the other ingredients. It gives the baked products tenderness and lightness, and as the sugar cooks it caramelizes, which gives the nicely browned appearance.

Sugar substitutes don't combine with other ingredients to make the product light and tender. They just contribute a sweetlike taste. They are valuable and useful in many recipes and certainly help to make the diabetic's menus much more interesting and varied without adding carbohydrates and calories. Unfortunately, they don't work well in baked foods because they undergo chemical changes in cooking and tend to become bitter rather than sweet. One of the challenges to food technologists is to develop an artificial sweetener that withstands heat.

You will note that a few of our recipes (Baked Custard, Bran Muffins, Birthday Cake) call for regular sugar. Sometimes the amount called for per serving is very small (Baked Custard) and adds only a few carbohydrates to the total nutrients, but is needed for sweetness and browning. In the case of the Birthday Cake and the Bran Muffins the sugar is needed for tenderness and lightness as well as taste. Please note the per serving nutrients and Food Exchanges. The sugar has been calculated into the total recipe and the Exchanges include the sugar as well as other ingredients used.

In any case, before you make any of the recipes calling for more than a tiny bit of sugar, we suggest you consult your doctor or diet counselor. If your diabetes condition is such that your body is especially sensitive to sucrose (sugar), you have, no doubt, already been advised to stay away from cakes and cookies. Your doctor may allow you to have an occasional small piece of the Birthday Cake if you and your diet counselor have calculated it into your day's menus.

However, no diabetics are allowed to sprinkle sugar on fruits or cereals or into beverages, and they are not permitted sweet desserts or regular soft drinks (except for emergency feedings as advised by diet counselors). And if you do include a food that has sugar in it, there is a definite need to know how much you can eat and the nutritive and Food Exchange values.

22

To Weigh Or Not to Weigh

So many times a newly diagnosed diabetic asks, "Do I have to buy special scales and weigh all of my food?" Well, some diabetics must certainly do this because their physicians have put them on a weighed diabetic diet.

Most diabetics, however, are on the Food Exchange system, which uses both weights (for meats) and measures (for the other food groups). So you will need a scale which measures food in grams, a set of standard measuring spoons, a set of metal measuring cups for dry measures and a glass measuring cup to measure liquids. Without these few pieces of equipment, accuracy and good dietary control is impossible.

In developing the recipes for this book, we have weighed and measured every single ingredient. Then we converted weights into household measures so that cooking will be faster and easier for you. But cooking for the diabetic can never be by a handful of this and that, cook until it looks right, and eat until you are full! Ingredients must be carefully measured and portions should be measured or weighed before serving.

Any diabetic who has done this will agree entirely with the reasons behind this advice. *There is no other way possible for anyone to become thoroughly eye-wise in judging how much is "X" amount of any given food.* If you consistently and conscientiously measure and weigh your foods day after day, you no longer go by "guesstimates" but achieve a certain eye skill in judging amounts. This is invaluable when eating out! It helps you to select a greater variety and gives you confidence in managing your diabetic diet.

By the way, if the diabetic in the family is not the cook, these words are directed primarily to the diabetic. The diabetic needs to know everything about his diet, even though he doesn't cook his own meals.

IV

Recipes

23

About Our Recipes

Every recipe in this book has been kitchen-tested by the authors. Family members and friends have been willing, interested, and eager taste-testers. And when each recipe was finalized the nutritive values and Food Exchange values were calculated from the latest data sources. Many of the recipes were originally developed by Kay over her years of volunteer work with the Northern Affiliate of the American Diabetes Association, Inc. A few were published in recipe sheets, others were published by the Association in booklet form, "Eats and Treats for the Young Diabetic" (1974).

Many other recipes had their initial tests in the Home Economics Department of Mundelein College, Chicago, by students in the experimental foods classes. Further development of these recipes was continued by the authors.

A few recipes were "donated" by diabetics and diet counselors we know and love. Then we tested them again making sure that each met our standards for taste, texture, and appearance. Finally they were calculated using the newest food composition tables and nutrient data provided on labels and by food manufacturers. At this point, Mary's calculator became her best friend and constant companion. Together we tackled the task of determining the proper Food Exchange values for each recipe. Once again we reviewed each recipe to make sure that directions are very clear so that they will be a success in your home kitchen.

For each recipe a serving size is indicated. That portion is adequate for most diabetics, but nondiabetics, especially hearty eaters, will want more. Consider the appetites of your family members and guests when deciding how much of each recipe to prepare. The diabetic's portion should be measured.

Because of the concern about dietary fats and the current emphasis on planning meals with more polyunsaturated fats and less saturated fat, we have used margarine or vegetable oil instead of butter in almost all of the recipes. We also offer you lots of delicious desserts, fruit yogurts, and sweet spreads that diabetics have been asking for.

Because many diabetics are also on low-sodium diets, we have calculated the sodium value for each recipe. If you have been advised to limit your salt or sodium intake, follow the directions at the bottom of each recipe. If you are on a fat-modified or a sodium-restricted diet, your diet counselor should review this book with you. You will need additional information on your special diet, and the recipes will be in addition to those instructions. If you are on a fat-modified diet, your counselor can easily mark this book to omit the High-Fat Meats and saturated fat foods that you should avoid.

24

Appetizers and Dips

Eggs a la Russe

Simple but so elegant! Mary's guests enjoy this one.

4 servings   1 serving: 2 egg halves plus 1½ tablespoons dressing

4 large eggs, hard-cooked
6 tablespoons Thousand Island Dressing (*see* Index)
¼ teaspoon coarsely ground pepper
1 rounded teaspoon caviar or 1 teaspoon chopped, ripe olives
4 leaves Boston or bibb lettuce
4 sprigs parsley

Remove shells from hard-cooked eggs; cut eggs in half lengthwise. Add pepper to Thousand Island Dressing. On serving plates arrange two egg halves (cut side down) on small lettuce leaf. Top with 1½ tablespoons Thousand Island Dressing. Garnish top of each with ¼ teaspoon of caviar and a sprig of parsley.

Nutritive values per serving: CHO 2 gm., PRO 8 gm., FAT 7 gm., Calories 102, Sodium 238 mg.

Food Exchange per serving: 1 High-Fat Meat Exchange.

Low-sodium diets: Omit salt in the Thousand Island Dressing recipe.

Eggplant Caviar

9 servings (yield: 2¼ cups)   1 serving: ¼ cup

2 medium (¾ pound each) eggplants
½ cup finely chopped onion
3 cloves garlic, minced
1 tablespoon lemon juice
2 tablespoons olive oil
½ cup chopped fresh parsley
1 teaspoon salt
¾ teaspoon coarsely ground pepper

Preheat oven to 350° F. (180° C.). Bake whole eggplants for 1 hour, or until tender, turning them occasionally. Peel off dark skin; mince the pulp. Stir in all other ingredients; mix well. Chill in covered bowl for several hours before using. Serve on crisp lettuce as a first course or mounded on melba toast as an hors d'oeuvre. Be sure to add the value of the melba toast (8 rounds = 1 Bread Exchange)

Nutritive values per serving: CHO 5 gm., PRO 1 gm., FAT 3 gm., Calories 49, Sodium 240 mg.

Food Exchanges per serving: 1 Vegetable Exchange plus ½ Fat Exchange. Up to 1½ tablespoons may be considered "free."

Low-sodium diets: Omit salt. Serve on lettuce or unsalted melba toast.

Eggplant Provençal

This very special dish of Mary's can be served as a first course or as a salad.

4 servings   1 serving: 1 piece of eggplant plus ¼ cup sauce

1 cup Real Italian Sauce (*see* Index), chilled
¼ teaspoon coarsely ground pepper
1 pound (1 medium or 2 small) eggplant
2 tablespoons Low-Calorie Italian Style Dressing (*see* Index)
4 lettuce leaves
1 tablespoon snipped parsley
1 teaspoon drained capers (optional)
Lettuce to line plates

Preheat oven to 350° F. (180° C.). Mix Real Italian Sauce with pepper and chill. Slice hard top off eggplant but leave skin on and cut lengthwise (if using small eggplants slice them in half, if using medium eggplant slice in quarters lengthwise). Pierce eggplant top and through skin several times with a fork. Brush eggplant all over with the Low-Calorie Italian Style Dressing; place in a baking pan. Bake 25 to 30 minutes, turning and basting after 15 minutes. Chill eggplant. When ready to serve line plates with lettuce, add a piece of eggplant, top with ¼ cup chilled Real Italian Sauce and sprinkle with snipped parsley and a few capers.

Nutritive values per serving: CHO 10 gm., PRO 2 gm., FAT 1 gm., Calories 51, Sodium 287 mg.

Food Exchanges per serving: 2 Vegetable Exchanges *or* 1 Fruit Exchange.

Low-sodium diets: Modify Real Italian Sauce recipe and Low-Calorie Italian Style Dressing recipe as directed.

Cocktail Meatballs

20 servings (yield: 80 meatballs)   1 serving: 4 tiny balls

1 pound very lean ground beef
1 large egg, beaten
¼ cup condensed beef broth
¼ teaspoon nutmeg
¼ teaspoon allspice
1 teaspoon grated lemon rind
4 teaspoons lemon juice
1 teaspoon salt
1 slice fresh bread, finely crumbled
2 tablespoons finely chopped onion

Preheat oven to 400° F. (205° C.). Prepare a shallow baking pan with vegetable pan coating (spray or solid); set it aside. Combine all ingredients; mix well. Form into tiny balls, measuring 1 level teaspoonful per ball. Place balls 1 inch apart in pan. Bake 10 minutes.

Nutritive values per serving: CHO 2 gm., PRO 5 gm., FAT 3 gm., Calories 54, Sodium 153 mg.

Food Exchange per serving: 1 Lean Meat Exchange.

Low-sodium diets: Omit salt. Substitute water for beef broth.

Soused Scallops

8 servings   1 serving: 4 to 5 pieces

1 package (12 ounces) frozen scallops
½ cup cider vinegar
¼ cup water
1½ teaspoons mixed pickling spices
1 tablespoon finely cut onion
½ teaspoon salt
Lettuce to line plates

Preheat oven to 350° F. (180° C.). Separate scallops and spread in small baking dish. Combine all remaining ingredients and pour over scallops. Cover and bake 15 minutes. Chill in liquid. Drain and serve on lettuce leaf.

Nutritive values per serving: CHO 5 gm., PRO 7 gm., FAT 3 gm., Calories 81, Sodium 242 mg.

Food Exchanges per serving: 1 Lean Meat Exchange plus ½ Fruit Exchange.

Low-sodium diets: This recipe is not suitable.

Stuffed Cherry Tomatoes

8 servings (yield: 32 tomatoes)   1 serving: 4 stuffed tomatoes

1 pound (about 32) cherry tomatoes, 1 inch in diameter
¾ cup Cheddar Cheese Dip or Curry Dressing or Dip (*see* Index)
2 tablespoons minced, fresh parsley

Slice tops off cherry tomatoes; gently scoop seed centers from tomatoes. Fill each with 1 teaspoon of dip or dressing. Sprinkle tops with parsley.

Nutritive values per serving:
    Cheddar Cheese Dip—CHO 3 gm., PRO 2 gm., FAT 1 gm., Calories 31, Sodium 106 mg.
    Curry Dressing—CHO 3 gm., PRO 1 gm., FAT 1 gm., Calories 18, Sodium 55 mg.

Food Exchange per serving: 1 Vegetable Exchange.

Low-sodium diets:
    Omit salt in Cheddar Cheese Dip or Curry Dressing.

Whipped Cottage Cheese

This is a base for many of our dips, but it is also delicious atop a baked potato.

9 servings (yield: 1 cup plus 2 tablespoons)   1 serving: 2 tablespoons

1 cup creamed cottage cheese
¼ cup water
⅛ teaspoon salt
1 tablespoon white vinegar

Combine all ingredients in a blender, cover tightly, and whip at low speed for 30 seconds or until smooth. Chill at least 2 hours before serving. If using this as a dip base, add other ingredients before chilling.

Nutritive values per serving: CHO 1 gm., PRO 3 gm., FAT 1 gm.,
Calories 21, Sodium 56 mg.

Food Exchange per serving: ½ Lean Meat Exchange.

Low-sodium diets: Omit salt.

Cheddar Cheese Dip

10 servings (yield: 1¼ cups)   1 serving: 2 tablespoons

2 ounces sharp Cheddar cheese, grated (about ½ cup)
1 cup (8 ounces) plain, low-fat yogurt
1 tablespoon minced parsley
½ teaspoon salt

Combine all ingredients; chill in a covered container 2 to 3 hours before serving.

Nutritive values per serving: CHO 1 gm., PRO 2 gm., FAT 2 gm.,
Calories 34, Sodium 158 mg.

Food Exchanges per serving: ½ Medium-Fat Meat Exchange. One
tablespoon may be considered "free."

Low-sodium diets: Omit salt.

Cheese and Onion Dip

12 servings (yield: 1¼ cups)   1 serving: 2 tablespoons

1 cup 2 tablespoons Whipped Cottage Cheese (*see* Index)
4 tablespoons finely cut green onions
5 tablespoons grated Parmesan cheese
Dash of cayenne pepper

Combine all ingredients, mix well, and chill at least 2 hours before serving.

Nutritive values per serving: CHO 1 gm., PRO 3 gm., FAT 1 gm.,
Calories 28, Sodium 109 mg.

Food Exchange per serving: ½ Lean Meat Exchange.

Low-sodium diets: This recipe is suitable.

Tangy Dill Dip

6 to 8 servings (yield: 1 cup)   1 serving: 3 tablespoons

1 cup (8 ounces) plain, low-fat yogurt
¼ teaspoon dried dill weed or 1 teaspoon chopped, fresh dill
¼ teaspoon salt
¼ teaspoon pepper

Combine all ingredients and chill in covered container 2 to 3 hours before serving.

Nutritive values per serving: CHO 2 gm., PRO 1 gm., FAT 1 gm.,
Calories 21, Sodium 121 mg.

Food Exchange per serving: Up to 3 tablespoons may be considered "free."

Low-sodium diets: Omit salt.

Harlequin Dip

Zippy dip for chunks of cooked meat, fish, or raw vegetables.

10 servings (yield: 1¼ cups)   1 serving: 2 tablespoons

1 cup (8 ounces) plain, low-fat yogurt
¼ cup chili sauce
1 tablespoon prepared horseradish, drained
1 teaspoon grated lemon rind
2 tablespoons finely cut celery
1 tablespoon finely cut green pepper
1 tablespoon finely cut green onion
½ teaspoon salt

Combine all ingredients well. Chill in a covered container 6 to 8 hours before serving.

Nutritive values per serving: CHO 3 gm., PRO 1 gm., FAT 1 gm.,
Calories 20, Sodium 204 mg.

Food Exchange per serving: Up to 2 tablespoons may be considered "free."

Low-sodium diets: Omit salt. Substitute dietetic, low-sodium catsup for chili sauce.

Horseradish Dip

10 servings (yield: 1¼ cups)   1 serving: 2 tablespoons

1 cup plus 2 tablespoons Whipped Cottage Cheese (*see* Index)
2 tablespoons prepared horseradish
2 tablespoons finely cut green pepper
¼ teaspoon dried basil
¼ teaspoon crushed, dried marjoram
¼ teaspoon salt
Dash of cayenne pepper

Combine all ingredients, mix well, and chill at least 2 hours before serving. Serve as a dip for raw vegetables or cooked ham cubes on toothpicks.

Nutritive values per serving: CHO 1 gm., PRO 3 gm., FAT 1 gm., Calories 23, Sodium 168 mg.

Food Exchange per serving: ½ Lean Meat Exchange for dip only.

Low-sodium diets: Omit salt.

West Indies Dip

Delightful as a dressing for a fresh fruit plate or with sliced apples, oranges, or bananas.

10 servings (yield: 1¼ cups)   1 serving: 2 tablespoons

1 cup plus 2 tablespoons Whipped Cottage Cheese (*see* Index)
1 tablespoon chopped onion
3 tablespoons chutney
1 teaspoon curry powder
⅛ teaspoon nutmeg

Combine all ingredients in a blender and cover tightly. Blend at low speed about 30 seconds or until smooth. Chill at least 2 hours before serving.

Nutritive values per serving: CHO 5 gm., PRO 3 gm., FAT 1 gm., Calories 35, Sodium 122 mg.

Food Exchange per serving: 1 Vegetable Exchange.

Low-sodium diets: This recipe is suitable.

Dip for Dawgs

This dip is especially good with cocktail "dawgs," tiny franks, or even for raw vegetable snacks.

8 servings (yield: 1 cup)   1 serving: 2 tablespoons

1 cup plain, low-fat yogurt
1 tablespoon prepared horseradish
1 tablespoon prepared mustard
¼ teaspoon salt
Few drops hot pepper sauce
Finely minced parsley (optional)

Combine all ingredients; blend well. Chill in a covered bowl for a few hours. For serving, garnish with a sprinkle of finely minced parsley.

Nutritive values per serving: CHO 2 gm., PRO 1 gm., FAT 0,
                    Calories 12, Sodium 107 mg.

Food Exchanges per serving: Up to 2 tablespoons may be considered
                    "free."

Low-sodium diets: Omit salt. Dip only vegetables, not franks.

25

Soups

Hearty Vegetable Soup

4 servings (yield: 4 cups)   1 serving: 1 cup

3½ cups boiling water
2 chicken bouillon cubes
2 beef bouillon cubes
1 can (16 ounces) tomatoes
½ cup chopped onions
½ cup thinly sliced carrots
½ cup slant-sliced celery
½ cup coarsely chopped green pepper
½ teaspoon salt
1 tablespoon lemon juice
5 whole peppercorns
½ teaspoon crushed sage
½ teaspoon hot pepper sauce

Combine all ingredients in a 3- to 4-quart pot. Bring to a boil, stirring to dissolve bouillon cubes. Cover and simmer gently for 1 hour. Stir occasionally to break up tomatoes into bite-sized pieces.

Nutritive values per serving: CHO 10 gm., PRO 3 gm., FAT 0,
                              Calories 51, Sodium 1,405 mg.

Food Exchanges per serving: 2 Vegetable Exchanges.

Low-sodium diets: Omit salt. Substitute low-sodium bouillon cubes and low-sodium canned tomatoes. Add 1 teaspoon basil.

Quick French Onion Soup

6 servings (yield: 6 cups)   1 serving: 1 cup

6 beef bouillon cubes
5 cups boiling water
3 tablespoons Worcestershire sauce
2 cups sliced onion rings
6 small rounds melba toast
3 tablespoons grated Parmesan cheese

Dissolve bouillon cubes in boiling water. Add Worcestershire sauce and onions. Cover and simmer gently for 25 to 30 minutes. Serve in warmed bowls with 1 melba toast round plus 1½ teaspoon Parmesan cheese sprinkled on top of each.

Nutritive values per serving: CHO 6 gm., PRO 3 gm., FAT 1 gm., Calories 52, Sodium 1303 mg.

Food Exchanges per serving: 1 Vegetable Exchange plus ½ Low-Fat Meat Exchange.

Low-sodium diets: Substitute unsalted beef bouillon cubes, low-sodium Worcestershire sauce, and unsalted melba toast.

Greek Egg-Lemon Soup

4 servings (yield: 2⅔ cups)   1 serving: ⅔ cup

4 chicken bouillon cubes
4 cups boiling water
2 tablespoons raw rice
2 medium eggs, beaten
2 tablespoons lemon juice
¼ teaspoon mixed herb seasoning
Dash of coarsely ground black pepper
Parsley

Dissolve bouillon cubes in boiling water; add rice slowly so as not to stop the boiling. Cover, turn heat low, let simmer gently for 15 minutes or until rice is tender but firm. Combine eggs and lemon juice. Slowly pour half of hot mixture into egg mixture, stirring quickly. Return to remaining soup and cook over very low heat 3 to 4 minutes, stirring continually, until mixture is smooth and coats the spoon. (Avoid boiling or high heat to prevent curdling.) Stir in herb seasoning and pepper. Spoon into bowls, garnish with parsley, and serve immediately.

Nutritive values per serving: CHO 6 gm., PRO 4 gm., FAT 3 gm., Calories 65, Sodium 987 mg.

Food Exchanges per serving: ½ Bread Exchange plus ½ Medium-Fat Meat Exchange.

Low-sodium diets: Substitute low-sodium chicken bouillon cubes.

Mushroom Vegetable Soup

A mushroom-picker's delight! Served with cheese and fruit, this hearty and delicious soup will make a full meal.

6 servings (yield: 6 cups)   1 serving: 1 cup

1 pound fresh mushrooms
2 tablespoons margarine
1 cup finely chopped carrots
1 cup finely chopped celery
1 cup finely chopped onions
1 clove garlic, minced
1 can (13¾ ounces) condensed beef broth
2 cups water
¼ cup tomato paste
2 tablespoons parsley flakes or ¼ cup minced fresh parsley
1 bay leaf
½ teaspoon salt
¼ teaspoon pepper
2 tablespoons dry sherry

Wash mushrooms; slice half of them and set aside. Chop remaining mushrooms and sauté them in 1 tablespoon margarine in a large pot. Add all the vegetables (except the sliced mushrooms) and cook 6 to 7 minutes, stirring often. Stir in all other ingredients except the mushrooms, the remaining margarine, and the sherry. Simmer, covered, for 1 hour. Puree soup in a blender. Sauté the sliced mushrooms in the remaining 1 tablespoon margarine. Return pureed soup to pot, add sautéed mushrooms and sherry. Reheat over moderate heat, stirring.

Nutritive values per serving: CHO 14 gm., PRO 6 gm., FAT 4 gm., Calories 124, Sodium 790 mg.

Food Exchanges per serving: 1 Bread Exchange plus ½ High-Fat Meat Exchange.

Low-sodium diets: This recipe is not suitable.

Zucchini Soup

4 servings (yield: 4 cups)   1 serving: 1 cup

1 tablespoon margarine
2 tablespoons finely chopped onion
1 clove garlic, crushed
1 pound young zucchini, cleaned and thinly sliced
2 tablespoons water
½ teaspoon curry powder
½ teaspoon salt
½ cup skim milk
1¾ cups chicken broth

Set a few slices of zucchini aside for garnish. Heat margarine in a heavy, deep skillet. Add onion, garlic, remainder of zucchini, and water. Cover and simmer gently for 10 minutes; stir with a wooden spoon while cooking. Remove from heat; add all remaining ingredients; mix well. Turn into blender and blend for 30 seconds. Serve hot or well chilled. Garnish each bowl with thin slices of zucchini.

Nutritive values per serving: CHO 7 gm., PRO 4 gm., FAT 3 gm., Calories 68, Sodium 670 mg.

Food Exchanges per serving: 1½ Vegetable Exchanges plus ½ Fat Exchange.

Low-sodium diets: Omit salt. Substitute unsalted margarine and low-sodium chicken broth.

Chicken Giblet Vegetable Soup

Leftover chicken giblets (heart, liver, gizzard) make a great soup. Chicken heart and gizzard should always be cooked until tender before combining with other ingredients.

4 servings (yield: 4 cups)   1 serving: 1 cup

Uncooked giblets of a chicken
4½ cups cold water
1 teaspoon salt
⅛ teaspoon pepper
½ cup finely diced carrots
½ cup finely chopped onions
½ cup finely chopped celery and leaves
1 small can (6 ounces) tomato juice
1 tablespoon dried parsley
¼ teaspoon paprika
2 tablespoons quick-cooking oatmeal

Wash giblets and discard all fat pieces. Place in a large cooking pot with water and salt. Bring to a boil and simmer about 25 minutes. Add all other ingredients except the oatmeal; simmer soup gently about 30 minutes more. Remove giblets and chop in small pieces. Return giblets to soup; add oatmeal, stir, and simmer 5 minutes.

Nutritive values per serving: CHO 8 gm., PRO 6 gm., FAT 1 gm., Calories 64, Sodium 675 mg.

Food Exchanges per serving: ½ Lean Meat Exchange plus 1 Vegetable Exchange, *or* ½ Bread Exchange plus ½ Lean Meat Exchange.

Low-sodium diets: Omit salt. Substitute unsalted tomato juice.

Cream of Tomato Soup

4 servings (yield: 3 cups)   1 serving: ¾ cup

1 can (16 ounces) tomatoes
½ cup chopped onions
2 tablespoons tomato paste
1½ cups chicken broth
1 bay leaf
½ teaspoon salt
⅛ teaspoon pepper
¾ cup (6 ounces) evaporated 2% milk
1 tablespoon finely cut parsley for garnish

Cut tomatoes in bite-sized pieces and place with tomato liquid in a saucepan; add onions, tomato paste, chicken broth, bay leaf, salt, and pepper. Bring to a boil; simmer, uncovered, for 5 minutes. Cool about 15 minutes; then turn into blender. Cover; blend at low speed until well mixed. Meanwhile, heat milk but do not allow it to boil or burn. Combine tomato mixture and hot milk. Simmer, uncovered, stirring constantly only until hot enough to serve. Garnish with parsley.

Nutritive values per serving: CHO 13 gm., PRO 6 gm., Fat 1 gm.,
Calories 85, Sodium 807 mg.

Food Exchange per serving: 1 Milk Exchange.

Low-sodium diets: This recipe is not suitable.

Crème Vichyssoise

This soup is delicious either hot or chilled but is usually served chilled.

4 servings (yield: 3 cups)   1 serving: ¾ cup

1 tablespoon vegetable oil
¼ cup finely chopped onion
1¾ cups chicken broth
1 cup skim milk
½ cup Half and Half
½ teaspoon salt
¼ teaspoon coarsely ground black pepper
1 cup (45 grams) dehydrated potato flakes, firmly packed
1 tablespoon finely chopped parsley for garnish

Heat vegetable oil in a large saucepan. Add onions and stir over medium heat until soft and tender but translucent. Add chicken broth; simmer 3 to 4 minutes. Add skim milk and Half and Half, and bring just to a low boil, stirring constantly. Remove from heat. Add salt, pepper, and potato flakes. Stir vigorously until dissolved and blended. Turn into a quart jar, cover, and chill a few hours before serving. Stir well before serving and garnish servings with finely chopped parsley.

Nutritive values per serving: CHO 16 gm., PRO 6 gm., FAT 7 gm., Calories 147, Sodium 639 mg.

Food Exchanges per serving: 1 Bread Exchange plus 1 High-Fat Meat Exchange.

Low-sodium diets: Omit salt. Substitute unsalted chicken broth.

Chilled Tomato Madrilene

6 servings (yield: 3 cups)   1 serving: ½ cup

1½ tablespoons granulated gelatin
½ cup cold water
2 cups tomato juice
¾ cup beef broth
1 teaspoon Worcestershire sauce
2 tablespoons lemon juice
6 teaspoons plain, low-fat yogurt
3 paper-thin lemon slices, cut in half
1 tablespoon finely minced parsley

Soak gelatin in cold water. Combine tomato juice, beef broth, Worcestershire sauce, and lemon juice in a heavy saucepan. Heat until very hot; stir in gelatin until completely dissolved. Pour into a 9-by-9-inch pan rinsed in cold water. Cool, cover pan, and chill in the refrigerator for several hours. Cut into ½-inch cubes. To serve, pile cubes carefully into bouillon cups. Top each with 1 level teaspoon yogurt, garnish with ½ slice lemon, and sprinkle with minced parsley.

Nutritive values per serving: CHO 5 gm., PRO 3 gm., FAT 0, Calories 35, Sodium 322 mg.

Food Exchange per serving: 1 Vegetable Exchange.

Low-sodium diets: Substitute unsalted tomato juice, low-sodium broth, and low-sodium Worcestershire sauce.

Cucumber Soup

A delicious cold soup for hot weather.

4 servings (yield: 3 cups)   1 serving: ¾ cup

1 pound (2 to 3) cucumbers, slender and firm
1¾ cups buttermilk, made from skim milk
1 teaspoon salt
1 teaspoon lemon juice
1 teaspoon finely minced onion
Paprika for garnish

Remove ends of cucumbers. Pare one, then slice into ¼-inch slices. If skins feel waxy, pare all cucumbers. Reserve 4 of the unpared slices for garnish, cut them again to yield 8 very thin slices; wrap and store in refrigerator. Pour ¼ cup buttermilk into blender; add half the cucumber slices. Blend at high speed for 30 to 40 seconds, until smooth. Add remaining cucumber slices, salt, lemon juice, and onion; blend about 1 minute. Stir in remaining buttermilk to mix thoroughly. Turn into a 1-quart jar, cover, and chill in refrigerator for at least 2 hours. (Do not keep longer than 48 hours before using.) Garnish each serving with thin slices of cucumber and a sprinkling of paprika.

Nutritive values per serving: CHO 9 gm., PRO 5 gm., FAT 0, Calories 56, Sodium 679 mg.

Food Exchanges per serving: 2 Vegetable Exchanges *or* ½ Milk Exchange plus ½ Vegetable Exchange.

Low-sodium diets: Omit salt. Substitute skim milk for buttermilk and increase lemon juice to 1 tablespoon. Add ½ teaspoon dill weed.

Fish Chowder

Because bacon burns easily, be sure to cook it over low or moderate heat.

6 servings (yield: 6 cups)   1 serving: 1 cup

1 pound fish fillets, fresh or frozen
4 thin slices bacon
¾ cup chopped onion
1 can (16 ounces) tomatoes
2 cups boiling water
1 cup diced, raw potatoes
½ cup diced carrots
½ cup finely chopped celery and leaves
⅓ cup catsup
2 teaspoons Worcestershire sauce
1 teaspoon salt
¼ teaspoon coarsely ground black pepper
⅛ teaspoon thyme
⅛ teaspoon marjoram
1 tablespoon minced parsley

Thaw frozen fish fillets. Remove bones and skin from fish; cut fish into 1-inch pieces. Cut bacon into ½-inch pieces. In a large saucepan over moderate heat, fry bacon until crisp, turning frequently. Add onions, and cook and stir over moderate heat until tender and translucent. Cut tomatoes in bite-sized pieces. Add tomatoes, tomato liquid from can, and all remaining ingredients except the fish and the parsley to the onions. Bring to a boil, turn heat low; cover and simmer for about 45 minutes. Add fish; cover and simmer for another 10 to 12 minutes, until fish flakes and is tender. Garnish each serving with a sprinkle of parsley.

Nutritive values per serving: CHO 15 gm., PRO 17 gm., FAT 5 gm., Calories 168, Sodium 772 mg.

Food Exchanges per serving: 1 Bread Exchange plus 2 Lean Meat Exchanges.

Low-sodium diets: Omit salt. Omit bacon. Use unsalted canned tomatoes, low-sodium catsup, and low-sodium Worcestershire sauce.

Gazpacho

9 servings (yield: 6¾ cups)   1 serving: ¾ cup

1 clove garlic, peeled
1 pound ripe tomatoes
1½ pounds (about 2 large) cucumbers
1 cup finely diced green pepper
¾ cup finely diced celery
½ cup finely diced onion
2 cups tomato juice or V-8 Juice
1 tablespoon vegetable oil
1 cup cold water
3 dashes Tabasco sauce
1 teaspoon salt
½ teaspoon coarsely ground pepper
½ cup seasoned croutons
Chopped parsley for garnish

Crush garlic into the bottom of a 2½-quart bowl. Core tomatoes and discard cores and seeds; finely dice tomatoes. Pare cucumbers, cut lengthwise in eighths, discard centers and seeds; finely dice remaining cucumber. Measure all ingredients except parsley and croutons into the large bowl on top of garlic. Mix thoroughly. Cover bowl tightly and chill for 2 hours or longer. Serve soup in chilled bowls garnished with croutons and parsley.

Nutritive values per serving: CHO 10 gm., PRO 2 gm., FAT 2 gm., Calories 57, Sodium 410 mg.

Food Exchanges per serving: 2 Vegetable Exchanges.

Low-sodium diets: Omit salt. Substitute unsalted tomato juice for V-8 or tomato juice.

26
Salads and Dressings

Bright Bean Salad

4 servings (yield: 2 cups)   1 serving: ½ cup

1 package (9 ounces) frozen French-cut green beans
1 medium carrot, finely chopped (2 ounces)
2 tablespoons finely chopped onion
⅛ teaspoon salt
3 tablespoons Lemon Shaker Dressing *(see* **Index)**

Cook green beans according to package directions, but reduce cooking time by 2 minutes so that beans are crisp. Drain beans and toss with chopped carrot, onion, salt, and dressing. Chill in a covered container for several hours.

Nutritive values per serving: CHO 6 gm., PRO 1 gm., FAT 0,
Calories 25, Sodium 230 mg.

Food Exchange per serving: 1 Vegetable Exchange.

Low-sodium diets: Omit salt in water in which beans are cooked and also in the Lemon Shaker Dressing.

Confetti Bean Salad

6 servings (yield: 3 cups)   1 serving: ½ cup

1 can (16 ounces) mixed cut green and wax beans
½ cup cider vinegar
1 teaspoon mixed pickling spices
½ cup finely diced celery
¼ cup chopped green pepper
¼ cup chopped onions
2 tablespoons chopped pimientos
Artificial sweetener to substitute for 5 teaspoons sugar
Crisp lettuce leaves

Drain beans, saving liquid. Combine this liquid with vinegar in a saucepan. Add mixed pickling spices, either loose or in a small cheesecloth bag. Bring to a boil, cover, turn heat to low, and simmer gently for 10 minutes. Meanwhile, mix all the vegetables in a bowl. Remove liquid from heat; add sweetener and stir until dissolved. Pour over vegetables and remove spice bag or loose spices. Chill several hours, stirring occasionally. Drain before serving on crisp lettuce.

Nutritive values per serving: CHO 5 gm., PRO 1 gm., FAT 0,
Calories 19, Sodium 120 mg.

Food Exchange per serving: 1 Vegetable Exchange.

Low-sodium diets: Substitute equal amounts of low-sodium canned
beans.

Brussels Sprouts and Carrot Salad

Colorful and attractive, this is an unusual salad for a buffet.

5 servings (yield: 2½ cups)   1 serving: ½ cup

1 package (10 ounces) frozen Brussels sprouts
1 can (16 ounces) sliced carrots
½ cup Lemon Shaker Dressing (*see* Index)

Cook Brussels sprouts according to package directions until they are crisp but tender; drain. Drain **carrots** and put them in a bowl; add Brussels sprouts and Lemon **Shaker** Dressing; mix well. Cover and refrigerate 4 to 6 hours before using; stir occasionally.

Nutritive values per serving: CHO 9 gm., PRO 2 gm., Fat 0, Calories 41, Sodium 310 mg.

Food Exchanges per serving: 2 Vegetable Exchanges *or* 1 Fruit Exchange.

Low-sodium diets: Omit salt in cooking Brussels sprouts and in the dressing recipe.

Carrot and Raisin Salad

This salad is Mary's Dad's favorite.

9 servings (yield: 3 cups)   1 serving: ⅓ cup lightly packed

3 cups shredded carrots
½ cup Low-Calorie Cooked Dressing (*see* Index)
⅓ cup (1½-ounce box) seedless raisins
¼ teaspoon salt
Lettuce leaves
Artificial sweetener to substitute for 6 teaspoons sugar (optional)

Combine all ingredients thoroughly. Cover bowl. Chill 2 hours or longer before serving. Serve on crisp lettuce.

Nutritive values per serving: CHO 8 gm., PRO 1 gm., FAT 1 gm., Calories 40, Sodium 168 mg.

Food Exchange per serving: 1 Fruit Exchange.

Low-sodium diets: Omit salt and prepare the Low-Calorie Cooked Dressing without salt.

Cucumber Salad

5 servings (yield: 2½ cups)   1 serving: ½ cup

1 large cucumber, peeled
1 cup plain, low-fat yogurt
2 tablespoons vinegar
1½ teaspoons dried dill weed or 1 tablespoon fresh dill
1 clove garlic, crushed, or ½ teaspoon garlic powder
½ teaspoon salt
¼ teaspoon pepper

Slice cucumber lengthwise and remove seeds. Dice the cucumber and add remaining ingredients. Mix thoroughly and chill at least ½ hour before serving.

Nutritive values per serving: CHO 4 gm., PRO 2 gm., FAT 1 gm., Calories 31, Sodium 238 mg.

Food Exchange per serving: 1 Vegetable Exchange.

Low-sodium diets: Omit salt.

Israeli Salad

6 servings (yield: 6 cups)   1 serving: 1 cup

2 cups prepared cucumbers (about 2)
½ cup chopped green peppers
2 cups shredded lettuce
2 tablespoons finely cut green onions
¾ cup grated or shredded carrots
2 tablespoons finely cut parsley
1 cup diced fresh tomatoes (about 2 tomatoes)
¼ cup sliced radishes
1 tablespoon vegetable oil
3 tablespoons lemon juice
1 teaspoon salt
¾ teaspoon coarsely ground black pepper

Pare cucumbers, cut in halves lengthwise, and discard seeds and center pulp. Dice cucumber flesh and measure 2 cups. Put cucumbers in a large bowl, and add all other ingredients. Toss together with a large salad spoon and fork for a few minutes. Serve immediately.

Nutritive values per serving: CHO 6 gm., PRO 1 gm., FAT 2 gm., Calories 45, Sodium 370 mg.

Food Exchanges per serving: 1 Vegetable Exchange plus ½ Fat Exchange.

Low-sodium diets: Omit salt.

Jackstraw Salad

4 servings (yield: 3 cups)   1 serving: ¾ cup

1 medium (about 4 ounces) red apple
½ cup green pepper strips
½ cup thin celery sticks
¾ cup shredded cabbage
¼ cup thinly sliced onion rings
⅓ cup Poppy Seed Dressing (*see* Index)
Crisp lettuce leaves

Remove core and stem of apple; leave skin on. Cut apple crosswise into ¼-inch rings; cut each ring into thin sticks about ⅛ inch wide. Cut green pepper and celery in similar tiny strips. Combine all ingredients (except lettuce) in a large bowl and toss lightly to mix Poppy Seed Dressing thoroughly. Serve on crisp lettuce

Nutritive values per serving: CHO 7 gm., PRO 1 gm., FAT 0. Calories 29, Sodium 114 mg.

Food Exchange per serving: 1 Vegetable Exchange.

Low-sodium diets: Omit salt in dressing recipe.

Mushroom Delight

6 servings (yield: 3 cups)   1 serving: ½ cup

1 tablespoon vegetable oil
1 tablespoon lemon juice
1 tablespoon wine vinegar
¼ teaspoon salt
⅛ teaspoon coarsely ground pepper
½ teaspoon dry mustard powder
⅛ teaspoon garlic powder or 1 clove garlic, crushed
1 to 2 tablespoons finely cut dill pickle
12 ounces fresh mushrooms, finely sliced (about 4½ cups)
2 tablespoons snipped, fresh parsley
6 lettuce leaves

Place all ingredients except mushrooms, parsley, and lettuce in a small jar. Cover the jar and shake it well. Drizzle dressing over mushrooms and toss mushrooms gently so that dressing thoroughly coats them. Serve on lettuce leaves and garnish with snipped parsley.

Nutritive values per serving: CHO 3 gm., PRO 2 gm., FAT 2 gm., Calories 37, Sodium 121 mg.

Food Exchange per serving: 1 Vegetable Exchange.

Low-sodium diets: Omit salt.

Red Cabbage Salad

5 servings (yield: 4 cups)   1 serving: ¾ cup

¾ cup cider vinegar
¼ cup cold water
½ teaspoon salt
½ teaspoon crushed tarragon
Artificial sweetener to substitute for 4 teaspoons sugar
2 cups shredded red cabbage
1 cup finely cut celery
½ cup chopped onions

Combine vinegar, water, salt, and tarragon; heat almost to a boil.

Remove from heat, add artificial sweetener and stir to dissolve. Mix vegetables, then pour vinegar mixture on top. Toss gently several times to mix well. Cover bowl and chill for a few hours. Just before serving, toss gently again.

Nutritive values per serving: CHO 7 gm., PRO 1 gm., FAT 0, Calories 27, Sodium 255 mg.

Food Exchange per serving: 1 Vegetable Exchange.

Low-sodium diets: Omit salt.

Spinach Salad

Here's another "cover girl!"

10 servings (yield: 10 cups)   1 serving: 1 cup

¾ pound raw spinach
1 cup bean sprouts, fresh or canned and drained
1 can (8½ ounces) water chestnuts, drained and sliced
2 medium eggs, hard-cooked
1 cup Miracle Red "French" Dressing (*see* Index)
Artificial sweetener to substitute for 3 teaspoons sugar
1 tablespoon vegetable oil

Clean and wash spinach, remove and discard stems, and tear leaves into bite-sized pieces. Pat spinach dry with paper towels and put in a large salad bowl. Spread a layer of bean sprouts, then a layer of water chestnuts over spinach. Slice eggs and distribute across top of salad. Cover salad with a damp paper towel and refrigerate to chill salad. Meanwhile add artificial sweetener and vegetable oil to Miracle Red "French" Dressing; mix well. Pour dressing over salad and toss immediately before serving.

Nutritive values per serving: CHO 6 gm., PRO 3 gm., FAT 3 gm., Calories 53, Sodium 179 mg.

Food Exchanges per serving: 1 Vegetable Exchange plus ½ Fat Exchange.

Low-sodium diets: Modify dressing as directed in that recipe.

Christmas Vegetable Salad Mold

The use of 1 teaspoon of sugar in 6 servings is OK!

6 servings (yield: 3 cups)   1 serving: ½ cup

1 tablespoon granulated gelatin
½ cup cold water
1 cup chicken broth
¼ teaspoon salt
½ teaspoon dried dill weed
1 teaspoon sugar
1 cup plain, low-fat yogurt
½ cup finely cut green pepper
½ cup quartered and sliced radishes
¼ cup finely cut green onions
2 tablespoons snipped fresh parsley
Crisp lettuce leaves

Combine gelatin and cold water in a heavy saucepan. Slowly heat over low heat, stirring constantly until gelatin is clear and liquid. Add chicken broth, salt, dill weed, and sugar; mix well. Add slowly to yogurt; mix well. Chill until it is of the consistency of unbeaten egg whites. Fold in remaining ingredients except lettuce; mix carefully. Turn into one 3-cup mold or six ½-cup molds. Cover lightly with clear plastic wrap. Chill until set. Unmold on crisp lettuce.

Nutritive values per serving: CHO 4 gm., PRO 3 gm., FAT 1 gm., Calories 36, Sodium 233 mg.

Food Exchange per serving: 1 Vegetable Exchange.

Low-sodium diets: Omit salt. Substitute low-sodium chicken broth.

Tomato Aspic Salad

4 servings (yield: 2 cups)   1 serving: ½ cup

½ cup cold water
1 tablespoon granulated gelatin
1½ cups tomato juice or V-8 Juice
1½ teaspoons lemon juice or white vinegar
1 to 2 drops hot pepper sauce
½ teaspoon minced onion
Crisp lettuce
Green pepper strips

Measure cold water into a small saucepan; sprinkle gelatin on top. Stir over low heat 3 to 4 minutes, or until gelatin is completely dissolved. Remove from heat. Add tomato juice with other ingredients (except lettuce and green pepper). Mix well. Chill until it is the consistency of unbeaten egg whites. Turn carefully into four ½-cup molds. Chill until firm. Unmold on crisp lettuce, garnish with green pepper strips, and serve with Low-Calorie Cooked Dressing or Lemon Mayonnaise (*see* Index).

Nutritive values per serving: CHO 4 gm., PRO 2 gm., FAT 0,
Calories 24, Sodium 207 mg.

Food Exchange per serving: 1 Vegetable Exchange.

Low-sodium diets: Substitute unsalted tomato juice. Omit salt in dressing recipe.

Waldorf Salad Mold

5 servings (yield: 2½ cups)   1 serving: ½ cup

1 tablespoon granulated gelatin
¼ cup cold water
1 tablespoon grated lemon rind
1½ cups water
¼ cup lemon juice
Artificial sweetener to substitute for 7 teaspoons sugar
2 drops yellow food color
¼ teaspoon pure lemon flavor
1 cup plain, low-fat yogurt
¾ cup finely diced red skin apples, with skin
¼ cup finely diced celery
2 tablespoons finely chopped walnuts
Lettuce for plates

Soak gelatin in ¼ cup cold water. Add lemon rind to another 1½ cups water; bring to a boil and simmer gently for 5 minutes. Strain, then measure only 1 cup to use; add gelatin mixture, lemon juice, artificial sweetener, food color, and lemon flavor; mix well. Chill until of consistency of unbeaten egg whites. Fold carefully into yogurt; then fold in diced apples, celery, and walnuts. Mix carefully but well. Turn into a 2½-cup salad mold or into **five** ½-cup molds. Cover and chill until firmly set. Serve as a salad on crisp lettuce.

Nutritive values per serving: CHO 7 gm., PRO 3 gm., FAT 3 gm., Calories 61, Sodium 31 mg.

Food Exchanges per serving: ½ Milk Exchange plus ½ Fat Exchange.

Low-sodium diets: This recipe is suitable.

Cheese-Vegetable Cold Plate

4 servings   1 serving: ½ cup Cheese Sandwich
                                              Spread plus assorted vegetables

2 cups Cheese Sandwich Spread (*see* Index)
Leaf lettuce
½ cup thinly sliced cucumbers
2 medium tomatoes, quartered
4 stalks celery, cut into strips
1 cup cauliflowerets
½ cup small, canned beets

Prepare Cheese Sandwich Spread and allow it to chill until flavors
are well blended. Line plates with lettuce. Mound ½ cup of cheese
mixture in the center of each plate. Divide vegetables evenly on each
plate, surrounding cheese and arranging so that there is attractive
color contrast.

Nutritive values per serving: CHO 11 gm., PRO 15 gm., FAT 16
                    gm., Calories 240, Sodium 690 mg.

Food Exchanges per serving: 2 High-Fat Meat Exchanges plus 2
                    Vegetable Exchanges.

Low-sodium diets: Substitute cream-style cottage cheese with chives
                    for cheese spread and count as 2 Medium-Fat
                    Meat Exchanges plus 2 Vegetable *or* 1 Fruit
                    Exchange.

Chef's Tuna Salad

6 servings   1 serving: ½ cup tuna plus 2 tablespoons Curry Dressing

2 cans (7 ounces each) tuna in oil
1 can (14½ ounces) asparagus pieces, drained
½ medium head lettuce, separated
¾ cup Curry Dressing or Dip (*see* Index)
3 hard-cooked eggs, sliced
Paprika

Chill canned tuna and asparagus. Drain tuna and flake lightly. Drain asparagus pieces well. Arrange lettuce on 6 salad plates. On each salad plate, place ⅓ cup of cut asparagus and ½ cup flaked tuna. Cover with 2 tablespoons Curry Dressing; top with 3 slices hard-cooked egg. Garnish with a sprinkle of paprika.

Nutritive values per serving: CHO 4 gm., PRO 21 gm., FAT 8 gm., Calories 176, Sodium 569 mg.

Food Exchanges per serving: 2½ Low-Fat Meat Exchanges plus 1 Vegetable Exchange.

Low-sodium diets: Substitute low-sodium canned tuna and low-sodium canned asparagus. Omit salt from dressing recipe.

Tuna Cheese Salad

4 servings (yield: 2⅔ cup)   1 serving: ⅔ cup

1 can (7 ounces) tuna, packed in water
¼ pound American, Cheddar, or Colby cheese
1½ tablespoons finely cut sweet gherkins
½ cup finely cut celery
½ cup Skim Milk Mayonnaise (*see* Index)
Crisp lettuce
Few strips of green pepper

Drain tuna; flake with fork into small pieces. Cut cheese into ¼-inch cubes. Combine tuna, cheese, gherkins, celery, and Skim Milk

Mayonnaise; mix well. Cover bowl, chill one hour or longer. Serve on crisp lettuce, garnished with thin strips of green pepper.

Nutritive values per serving: CHO 4 gm., PRO 22 gm., FAT 10 gm., Calories 201, Sodium 508 mg.

Food Exchanges per serving: 3 Lean Meat Exchanges plus 1 Vegetable Exchange.

Low-sodium diets: Substitute low-sodium cheese. Omit salt in Skim Milk Mayonnaise.

Chicken Salad Deluxe

4 servings (yield: 4 cups)   1 serving: 1 cup

2 cups, firmly packed, cubed, cooked chicken
¼ cup chicken broth
1 cup slant-cut celery
2 tablespoons finely cut green onion
¼ cup thinly sliced green pepper
1 can (2 ounces) mushroom stems and pieces, drained
24 small (100 grams) Thompson seedless grapes
¼ cup slivered almonds
2 teaspoons margarine
¾ cup Low-Calorie Cooked Dressing (*see* Index)
Crisp lettuce leaves

In a large bowl combine cubed cooked chicken, chicken broth, celery, onions, green pepper, mushrooms, and grapes; mix well. Cover and chill several hours. Sauté the almonds in margarine, stirring constantly, until they are browned; spread on paper towel to cool. Immediately before serving stir the dressing into the chicken salad. Arrange chicken salad on four plates, lined with crisp lettuce leaves, and top each with one tablespoon of sautéed almonds.

Nutritive values per serving: CHO 8 gm., PRO 33 gm., FAT 11 gm., Calories 265, Sodium 473 mg.

Food Exchanges per serving: 1 Fruit Exchange plus 4½ Lean Meat Exchanges.

Low-sodium diets: Substitute unsalted margarine and broth. Omit salt in the Low-Calorie Cooked Dressing.

DRESSINGS

Buttermilk Mayonnaise

This buttermilk dressing is delicious served on mixed greens or sliced tomatoes. It is also an excellent sauce on some cooked vegetables or steamed or baked fish fillets.

8 servings (yield: 1 cup)   1 serving: 2 tablespoons

½ teaspoon granulated gelatin
1 tablespoon cold water
½ teaspoon dry mustard
¼ teaspoon salt
Few grains black pepper
1 tablespoon water
1 cup buttermilk, made from skim milk
2 teaspoons finely cut green onions
2 teaspoons minced parsley

Soak gelatin in 1 tablespoon cold water. Dissolve over hot water. Mix together mustard, salt, pepper, and 1 tablespoon water until smooth. Combine all ingredients except parsley and blend well. Chill until it begins to thicken. Beat gently until smooth; stir in parsley. Turn into a jar and cover. Chill several hours.

Nutritive values per serving: CHO 2 gm., PRO 1 gm., FAT 0,
                                    Calories 12, Sodium 107 mg.

Food Exchange per serving: Up to 2 tablespoons may be considered
                                    "free."

Low-sodium diets: Omit salt.

Buttermilk Salad Dressing

This dressing is delicious on vegetable salads.

10 servings (yield: 2 cups)   1 serving: 3 tablespoons

2 cups buttermilk, made from skim milk
¼ teaspoon black pepper
½ teaspoon garlic powder
½ teaspoon salt
½ teaspoon dried parsley flakes
¼ cup finely cut green onions

Mix all ingredients thoroughly. If available, use a blender set at low speed for 30 seconds. Turn into a pint jar, cover tightly, and store in refrigerator a few hours before using.

Nutritive values per serving: CHO 3 gm., PRO 2 gm., FAT 0,
Calories 18, Sodium 160 mg.

Food Exchange per serving: Up to 3 tablespoons may be considered "free."

Low-sodium diets: Omit salt.

Curry Dressing or Dip

This is easy and delicious as a dressing on chicken or fish salads or as a dip for assorted raw vegetables.

8 servings (yield: 1 cup)   1 serving: 2 tablespoons

1 cup plain, low-fat yogurt
½ teaspoon curry powder
⅛ teaspoon powdered ginger
¼ teaspoon salt
Dash of cayenne pepper

Blend all ingredients until smooth; chill in a covered container

Nutritive values per serving: CHO 1 gm., PRO 1 gm., FAT 0.5 gm.
Calories 14, Sodium 81 mg.

Food Exchange per serving: Up to 2 tablespoons may be considered
"free."

Low-sodium diets: Omit salt.

Lemon Mayonnaise

For fruit, chicken, or seafood salads.

12 servings (yield: 1½ cups)   1 serving: 2 tablespoons

1 tablespoon cornstarch
2 teaspoons dry mustard
1½ teaspoons salt
1 cup water
2 medium eggs, beaten
⅓ cup lemon juice
2 tablespoons white vinegar
Artificial sweetener to substitute for 6 teaspoons sugar

Combine cornstarch, mustard, and salt in the top of a double boiler. Combine water and beaten eggs. Slowly add to cornstarch mixture, stirring constantly, until smooth. Cook over simmering water for 5 minutes, stirring constantly. Very slowly stir in the lemon juice and vinegar. Continue cooking and stirring over simmering water for 10 more minutes. Remove from heat. Add the artificial sweetener; mix well. Pour into a pint jar; cover and store in refrigerator. Stir well before each use.

Nutritive values per serving: CHO 1 gm., PRO 1 gm., FAT 1 gm., Calories 17, Sodium 275 mg.

Food Exchange per serving: Up to 2 tablespoons may be considered "free."

Low-sodium diets: Omit salt.

Lemon Shaker Dressing

10 servings (yield: 1¼ cups)   1 serving: 2 tablespoons

½ cup lemon juice
¾ cup water
¼ teaspoon salt
1 teaspoon grated lemon rind
½ teaspoon Worcestershire sauce
¼ teaspoon celery seed
⅛ teaspoon black pepper
¼ teaspoon dry mustard
Artificial sweetener to substitute for 2 tablespoons sugar

Combine all ingredients in a pint jar; cover tightly and shake vigorously. Store in refrigerator. Shake before using.

Nutritive values per serving: CHO 1 gm., PRO 0, FAT 0, Calories 3, Sodium 63 mg.

Food Exchange per serving: Up to 3 tablespoons may be considered "free."

Low-sodium diets: Omit salt.

Low-Calorie Cooked Dressing

16 servings (yield: 1½ cups)   1 serving: 1½ tablespoons

⅓ cup instant nonfat dry milk
1¼ teaspoon dry mustard
1 teaspoon salt
⅛ teaspoon black pepper
1 tablespoon flour
1 medium egg
1 cup water
2 tablespoons white vinegar
1 tablespoon margarine
Artificial sweetener to substitute for 6 teaspoons sugar

Combine dry ingredients in the top of a double boiler. Beat egg slightly and combine with water and vinegar. Add to dry ingredients slowly, stirring to blend well. Cook over simmering water, stirring constantly until thick and smooth. Remove from heat. Add margarine and artificial sweetener; blend well. Turn into a pint jar; cover. Store in refrigerator.

Nutritive values per serving: CHO 1 gm., PRO 1 gm., FAT 1 gm.,
                              Calories 18, Sodium 153 mg.

Food Exchange per serving: Up to 1½ tablespoons may be
                           considered "free."

Low-sodium diets: Omit salt. Substitute unsalted margarine.

Low-Calorie Italian-Style Dressing

8 servings (yield: 1 cup)   1 serving: 2 tablespoons

⅔ cup tomato juice
1 tablespoon vegetable oil
⅓ cup wine vinegar
1 tablespoon Italian seasoning
$\frac{1}{16}$ teaspoon garlic powder or 1 small fresh garlic clove, crushed
¼ teaspoon salt

Measure all ingredients into a pint jar; cover. Shake vigorously. Store in refrigerator. Shake before using.

Nutritive values per serving: CHO 1 gm., PRO 0, FAT 2 gm., Calories 20, Sodium 108 mg.

Food Exchange per serving: Up to 2 tablespoons may be considered "free."

Low-sodium diets: Omit salt. Substitute unsalted tomato juice.

Miracle Red "French" Dressing

The miracle is that this delicious dressing is fat-free and will not use up your Fat Exchanges.

8 to 16 servings (yield: 1 cup)   1 serving: 1 to 2 tablespoons

½ teaspoon granulated gelatin
1 tablespoon cold water
¼ cup boiling water
½ teaspoon salt
½ cup tomato juice
¼ cup white vinegar
⅛ teaspoon garlic powder
Dash black pepper
¼ teaspoon dry mustard
½ teaspoon Worcestershire sauce
Artificial sweetener to substitute for 1 tablespoon sugar

Soften gelatin in cold water. Add boiling water; stir until dissolved. Turn into a pint jar with all the remaining ingredients. Cover tightly; shake thoroughly. Chill for a few hours before serving. Stir occasionally to prevent gelling at bottom. Shake gently before using.

Nutritive values per serving: CHO 1 gm., PRO 0, FAT 0, Calories 4, Sodium 176 mg.

Food Exchange per serving: Up to ¼ cup may be considered "free."

Low-sodium diets: Omit salt. Substitute unsalted tomato juice and low-sodium Worcestershire sauce.

Mustard Dressing

8 servings (yield· 1 cup)   1 serving: 2 tablespoons

1½ teaspoons dry mustard
1 tablespoon water
2 tablespoons flour
1 teaspoon salt
Dash of cayenne pepper
2 egg yolks, well beaten
¾ cup water
2 tablespoons white vinegar
Artificial sweetener to substitute for 3 teaspoons sugar

Mix mustard and 1 tablespoon water in a small container until smooth; let stand 5 minutes. Mix together flour, salt, and cayenne pepper in top of a double boiler. Combine beaten egg yolks, ¾ cup water, and mustard. Add to dry ingredients and mix well. Cook and stir over simmering water 10 minutes or until thick and smooth. Remove from heat. Add vinegar and artificial sweetener; blend well. Pour into ½-pint jar; cover and chill. Stir before using.

Nutritive values per serving: CHO 2 gm., PRO 1 gm., FAT 1 gm.,
                              Calories 20, Sodium 268 mg.

Food Exchange per serving: Up to 2 tablespoons may be considered
                           "free."

Low-sodium diets: Omit salt.

Mustard Yogurt Dressing

8 servings (yield: 1 cup)   1 serving: 2 tablespoons

1 cup plain, low-fat yogurt
1 teaspoon dry mustard
½ teaspoon paprika
1 teaspoon salt
1 teaspoon sugar (Don't worry, it's OK.)

Combine seasonings with ¼ cup of the yogurt; mix thoroughly. Add to remaining yogurt. Mix well, turn into a small jar, cover, and chill several hours before use.

Nutritive values per serving: CHO 2 gm., PRO 1 gm., FAT 0, Calories 16, Sodium 148 mg.

Food Exchange per serving: Up to 2 tablespoons may be considered "free."

Low-sodium diets: Omit salt.

No-Calorie Dressing

Kay is especially proud of this one—her diabetic friends rave about it!

8 to 16 servings (yield: 1 cup)   1 serving: 1 to 2 tablespoons

½ cup water
½ cup white vinegar
½ teaspoon salt
½ teaspoon dry mustard
⅛ teaspoon pepper
1/16 teaspoon paprika
Artificial sweetener to substitute for 4 teaspoons sugar

Combine all ingredients in a pint jar and cover tightly. Shake vigorously and store in refrigerator. Shake before using.

Nutritive values per serving: No CHO, PRO, FAT, or Calories in entire recipe.
Sodium value of 2 tablespoons is 133 mg.

Food Exchange per serving: This is a "free" dressing!

Low-sodium diets: Omit salt.

Poppy Seed Dressing

Follow recipe for No-Calorie Dressing, but use cider vinegar in place of white vinegar, omit paprika, and add 1 tablespoon poppy seeds. Delicious over fruit salads.

Skim Milk Mayonnaise

16 servings (yield: 2 cups)   1 serving: 2 tablespoons

1½ teaspoons granulated gelatin
¼ cup cold water
1½ cups skim milk
2 medium egg yolks, beaten
1½ teaspoons dry mustard
1 teaspoon salt
¼ teaspoon paprika
¼ cup white vinegar
Artificial sweetener to substitute for 3 teaspoons sugar

Soak gelatin in cold water; set aside. Scald milk in the top of a double boiler. Slowly pour over beaten yolks, stirring constantly to prevent curdling. Return egg-milk mixture to the top of the double boiler and add mustard, salt, and paprika. Cook over simmering water, stirring continually until mixture is thick enough to coat the spoon. Remove from heat. Add vinegar, gelatin, and artificial sweetener; blend well. Pour into a pint jar; cover and chill. Stir before using.

Nutritive values per serving: CHO 1 gm., PRO 1 gm., FAT 1 gm., Calories 16, Sodium 146 mg.

Food Exchange per serving: Up to 2 tablespoons may be considered "free."

Low-sodium diets: Omit salt.

Summer Dressing

8 servings (yield: 1½ cups)   1 serving: 3 tablespoons

1 cup plain, low-fat yogurt
½ cup finely chopped cucumber (seeds removed)
2 tablespoons finely chopped radishes
1 tablespoon minced, fresh parsley
1 tablespoon finely cut green onions
1 tablespoon lemon juice
1 tablespoon prepared horseradish
¼ teaspoon salt
Dash of cayenne pepper

Combine all ingredients and mix well. Refrigerate at least 2 hours before serving.

Nutritive values per serving: CHO 3 gm., PRO 1 gm., FAT 0, Calories 17, Sodium 84 mg.

Food Exchange per serving: Up to 3 tablespoons may be considered "free."

Low-sodium diets: Omit salt.

Thousand Island Dressing

6 to 12 servings (yield: ¾ cup)   1 serving: 1 to 2 tablespoons

½ cup Skim Milk Mayonnaise (*see* Index)
1½ tablespoons catsup or chili sauce
¼ cup finely cut dill pickle
2 tablespoons minced parsley
1 tablespoon minced green onion

Combine all ingredients thoroughly. Chill before using.

Nutritive values per serving: CHO 2 gm., PRO 1 gm., FAT 0.5 gm., Calories 16, Sodium 229 mg.

Food Exchange per serving: Up to 2 tablespoons may be considered "free."

Low-sodium diets: This recipe is not suitable.

27

Breads and Sandwiches

Baking Powder Biscuits

12 biscuits

1 serving: 1 biscuit

2 cups sifted flour
4 teaspoons baking powder
½ teaspoon salt
5 tablespoons margarine
¾ cup skim milk

Preheat oven to 425°F. (218°C.). Sift together flour, baking powder, and salt. Cut margarine in with a blending fork or dough blender until fat is the size of small peas. Add milk all at once. Stir until dough is all mixed and forms a ball. Roll out on a lightly floured board to a thickness of about ¼ inch. Cut with a 2½-inch round cutter. If thicker biscuits are desired, roll out to a thickness of ½ inch and cut with a 2-inch cutter, yielding 16 biscuits. Place 1 inch apart on a baking sheet. Bake 12 to 14 minutes.

Nutritive values per serving:
    2½-inch biscuit—   CHO 15 gm., PRO 3 gm., FAT 5 gm., Calories 118, Sodium 252 mg.

2-inch biscuit—	CHO 12 gm., PRO 2 gm., FAT 4 gm., Calories 89, Sodium 189 mg.
Food Exchanges per serving:	1 Bread Exchange plus 1 Fat Exchange.
Low-sodium diets:	Omit salt. Use low-sodium baking powder and unsalted margarine.

Buttermilk Biscuits

16 biscuits   1 serving: 1 biscuit

2 cups sifted flour
½ teaspoon salt
2 teaspoons baking powder
½ teaspoon baking soda
1 tablespoon sugar
5 tablespoons margarine
¾ cup buttermilk, made from skim milk

Preheat oven to 425°F. (218°C.). Sift together dry ingredients. Cut in margarine with a pastry blender or blending fork. Add buttermilk all at once; blend with a fork just until flour is moistened and dough pulls away from the sides of the bowl. Turn out onto a lightly floured board or wax paper. Knead lightly for 30 seconds. Roll out to a thickness of ½ inch. Cut with a 2-inch round cutter. If using a 2½-inch cutter, roll out to a thickness of ¼ inch and cut 16 biscuits. Place 1 inch apart on a baking pan. Bake 12 to 15 minutes.

Nutritive values per serving:

2½-inch biscuit—	CHO 17 gm., PRO 3 gm., FAT 5 gm., Calories 122, Sodium 267 mg.
2-inch biscuit—	CHO 12 gm., PRO 2 gm., FAT 4 gm., Calories 92, Sodium 200 mg.
Food Exchanges per serving:	1 Bread Exchange plus 1 Fat Exchange.
Low-sodium diets:	Omit salt and regular baking powder, substituting 4 teaspoons low-sodium baking powder; use unsalted margarine; substitute skim milk plus ¾ teaspoon vinegar for buttermilk.

Bran Muffins

9 muffins   1 serving: 1 muffin

1 cup All-Bran cereal
⅔ cup skim milk
½ cup sifted flour
1½ teaspoons baking powder
½ teaspoon salt
¼ cup sugar (Don't worry, it's OK.)
1 medium egg, beaten
2 tablespoons vegetable oil

Preheat oven to 400° F. (205° C.). Prepare nine 2-inch muffin cups with vegetable pan coating (spray or solid) or line with paper baking cups. Combine bran and milk. Sift together flour, baking powder, salt, and sugar. Combine beaten egg and vegetable oil; add to bran and milk; mix well. Add dry ingredients all at once and stir (do not beat) just enough to mix. Measure three scant tablespoonfuls batter into each of the nine prepared muffin cups. Bake 25 to 30 minutes. Cool 5 minutes, then turn out of pans.

Nutritive values per serving: CHO 17 gm., PRO 3 gm., FAT 4 gm., Calories 107, Sodium 237 mg.

Food Exchanges per serving: 1 Bread Exchange plus 1 Fat Exchange.

Low-sodium diets: Omit salt. Substitute low-sodium baking powder for regular baking powder.

Raisin Bran Muffins

To preceding Bran Muffin recipe add ¼ cup seedless raisins to the dry ingredients.

Nutritive values per serving of 1 muffin: CHO 20 gm., PRO 3 gm., FAT 4 gm., Calories 119, Sodium 238 mg.

Food Exchanges per serving of 1 muffin: 1 Bread Exchange plus ½ Fruit Exchange plus 1 Fat Exchange.

Corn Meal Muffins

12 muffins   1 serving: 1 muffin

1 cup yellow cornmeal
¾ cup sifted flour
½ teaspoon salt
1½ teaspoons baking powder
½ teaspoon baking soda
1 tablespoon sugar (Don't worry, it's OK.)
1 medium egg, beaten
1 cup buttermilk, made from skim milk
2 tablespoons margarine, melted

Preheat oven to 400° F. (205° C.). Prepare twelve 2½-inch muffin pans with vegetable pan coating (spray or solid) or line with paper baking cups. Sift together all dry ingredients and mix lightly with a fork. Combine beaten egg, buttermilk, and melted margarine; mix well. Add all at once to dry ingredients. Stir vigorously to mix well, then beat gently for 1 to 2 minutes. Fill prepared muffin pans half full (3 tablespoons batter per muffin). Bake for 25 to 30 minutes. Serve hot.

Nutritive values per serving: CHO 15 gm., PRO 3 gm., FAT 3 gm., Calories 94, Sodium 231 mg.

Food Exchanges per serving: 1 Bread Exchange plus ½ Fat Exchange.

Low-sodium diets: Omit salt, baking soda, and regular baking powder; substitute 2½ teaspoons low-sodium baking powder; use unsalted margarine; substitute skim milk plus 1 teaspoon vinegar for buttermilk.

Buttermilk Corn Bread

16 servings   1 serving: a 2-by-2-by-1-inch square

1 cup sifted flour
½ teaspoon baking soda
2 teaspoons baking powder
½ teaspoon salt
1 tablespoon sugar (Don't worry, its OK.)
1 cup yellow cornmeal
1 medium egg, beaten
1 cup buttermilk, made from skim milk
3 tablespoons margarine, melted

Preheat oven to 425° F. (218° C.). Prepare an 8-by-8-by-2-inch pan with vegetable pan coating (spray or solid). Sift together dry ingredients. Combine egg, buttermilk, and margarine, and add to dry ingredients, stirring until well mixed. Beat with a rotary beater for 1 minute. Turn into the prepared pan. Bake 20 to 25 minutes. Cool slightly, then cut into sixteen 2-inch squares. Serve warm.

Nutritive values per serving: CHO 12 gm., PRO 2 gm., FAT 3 gm., Calories 91, Sodium 200 mg.

Food Exchanges per serving: 1 Bread Exchange plus ½ Fat Exchange.

Low-sodium diets: Omit salt, regular baking powder and baking soda; substitute 4 teaspoons low-sodium baking powder; use unsalted margarine; substitute skim milk plus 1 teaspoon vinegar for buttermilk.

Corn Toasties

18 toasties   1 serving: 1 toastie

1 cup sifted flour
2 tablespoons sugar (Don't worry, it's OK.)
1½ teaspoons baking powder
½ teaspoon salt
½ teaspoon baking soda
2 cups yellow cornmeal
¾ cup buttermilk, made from skim milk
1 medium egg, beaten
2 tablespoons margarine, melted

Sift together flour, sugar, baking powder, salt, and baking soda. Stir dry ingredients into cornmeal. In another bowl, combine remaining ingredients and beat until frothy and well blended. Add all at once to dry ingredients; stir until well mixed. Turn onto a lightly floured board and knead only 10 times. Roll out to a thickness of ¼ inch; cut with a 3-inch-diameter cutter. Bake on a warm ungreased griddle or frying pan about 10 minutes on each side.

Nutritive values per serving: CHO 16 gm., PRO 2 gm., FAT 2 gm., Calories 92, Sodium 150 mg.

Food Exchanges per serving: 1 Bread Exchange plus ½ Fat Exchange.

Low-sodium diets: Omit salt, regular baking powder and baking soda; substitute 3 teaspoons low-sodium baking powder; use unsalted margarine; substitute skim milk plus ¾ teaspoon vinegar for buttermilk.

Yankee Johnny Cake

If you don't have buttermilk, substitute 1 cup of skim milk mixed with 1 teaspoon lemon juice or vinegar.

16 squares   1 serving: 1½-inch square

1 cup sifted flour
1 cup yellow cornmeal
1 teaspoon baking soda
½ teaspoon salt
Artificial sweetener to substitute for 1 tablespoon sugar
1 medium egg, beaten
1 cup buttermilk, made from skim milk
3 tablespoons vegetable oil

Preheat oven to 400° F. (205° C.). Prepare an 8-by-8-by-2-inch pan with vegetable pan coating (spray or solid). Sift together all dry ingredients. Combine egg and buttermilk and add to dry ingredients all at once; add oil. Stir (do not beat) just until dry ingredients are all moistened. Pour into the prepared pan and bake 25 to 30 minutes. Cut into sixteen 1½-inch squares.

Nutritive values per serving: CHO 13 gm., PRO 2 gm., FAT 3 gm., Calories 90, Sodium 167 mg.

Food Exchanges per serving: 1 Bread Exchange plus ½ Fat Exchange.

Low-sodium diets: Omit salt and baking soda. Use 2 teaspoons low-sodium baking powder and substitute skim milk mixed with 1 teaspoon lemon juice or vinegar for the buttermilk.

Popovers

If you want really puffed-up, high popovers, heat the custard cups or muffin pans before *you pour the batter in.*

8 popovers   1 serving: 1 popover

1 teaspoon vegetable oil (to oil pans)
2 medium eggs, beaten slightly
1 cup whole milk
1 cup sifted flour
½ teaspoon salt
2 teaspoons vegetable oil

Preheat oven to 475° F. (250° C.). Oil 8 custard cups or 2½-inch muffin pans with vegetable oil and set aside. Combine eggs, milk, flour, and salt and beat until frothy, about 1½ minutes. Add 2 teaspoons vegetable oil; beat only 30 seconds, no more. Pour batter into the custard cups or muffin pans. Bake 15 minutes; then reduce heat to 350° F. (180° C.) and bake for another 30 minutes, or until firm and browned. A few minutes before popovers are completely cooked, pierce top or side of each with a sharp knife to let the steam escape. If you prefer drier popovers, leave them in the oven with the oven door wide open for 20 minutes after the heat has been turned off.

Nutritive values per serving: CHO 12 gm., PRO 4 gm., FAT 4 gm., Calories 100, Sodium 162 mg.

Food Exchanges per serving: 1 Bread Exchange plus 1 Fat Exchange.

Low-sodium diets: Omit salt.

Bread Stuffing

This recipe may be made from any brand of dry Herb Stuffing Mix. The amount here is for a 5- to 8-pound roasting chicken or capon. For a 12- to 16-pound turkey, double the recipe. It is a truly delicious dressing, and for many people the butter and eggs will never be missed!

10 servings (yield: 5 cups)   1 serving: ½ cup

1 package (8 ounces) Herb Stuffing Mix
1 teaspoon grated lemon rind
1½ cups (scant) chicken broth, boiling

Combine all ingredients; mix well. Stuff and cook prepared bird.

Nutritive values per serving: CHO 17 gm., PRO 3 gm., FAT 1 gm., Calories 87, Sodium 412 mg.

Food Exchange per serving: 1 Bread Exchange.

Low-sodium diets: This recipe is not suitable.

Cinnamon Sweet Roll

1 serving   1 serving: 1 roll

1 slice soft white bread
1 tablespoon cream-style cottage cheese
½ teaspoon sugar (Don't worry, it's OK.)
⅟₁₆ teaspoon cinnamon
⅛ teaspoon pure vanilla
10 seedless raisins

Roll bread with a rolling pin until flat. Mash together the cheese, sugar, cinnamon, and vanilla. Spread cheese mixture on bread; scatter raisins across center only. Roll like a jelly roll and fasten with toothpicks. Broil 3 to 4 inches below broiler until lightly toasted.

Nutritive values per serving: CHO 19 gm., PRO 4 gm., FAT 1 gm., Calories 101, Sodium 175 mg.

Food Exchanges per serving: 1 Bread Exchange plus ½ Fruit Exchange.

Low-sodium diets: Substitute low-sodium bread.

California Sunshine Bread

If the water or orange juice are very hot the yeast will be destroyed. If the liquid is too cold the yeast action will be too slow.

20 slices (yield: 1¼-pound loaf)   1 serving: 1-ounce slice (28 grams)

¼ cup lukewarm water (110° to 115° F. or 43° to 46° C.)
3 tablespoons sugar (Don't worry, it's OK.)
1 package instant active dry yeast
⅔ cup fresh orange juice (warmed to room temperature)
2½ cups unsifted white flour
1 teaspoon salt
3 tablespoons margarine, melted
1 tablespoon finely grated fresh orange rind
1 teaspoon finely grated fresh lemon rind
2 teaspoons vegetable oil (to oil pans)

Combine lukewarm water, sugar, and dry yeast in a large bowl, stirring until completely dissolved. Add warm orange juice and beat until well blended. Add 1 cup of the flour gradually, beating gently until smooth. Cover bowl and set in a warm place until bubbly and light (30 to 40 minutes). Add salt, margarine, grated orange and lemon rinds, and beat gently to mix. Stir in remaining flour gradually, mixing well. Turn onto a lightly floured board and knead until smooth and elastic (about 10 minutes). Place in a large, oiled bowl, turning dough around to coat all over. Cover bowl; place in a warm place until dough has doubled in size (1 to 2 hours). Punch dough down in several places. Knead on board for 5 minutes. Shape into a loaf and place in an oiled 8½-by-4½-by-2½-inch loaf pan. Cover, let rise in a warm place about 1 hour. Preheat oven to 375° F. (190° C.). When bread has risen, bake 35 to 45 minutes.

Nutritive values per serving: CHO 15 gm., PRO 2 gm., FAT 2 gm., Calories 88, Sodium 128 mg.

Food Exchanges per serving: 1 Bread Exchange plus ½ Fat Exchange.

Low-sodium diets: Omit salt. Use unsalted margarine.

Dilly Bread

22 slices (yield: 22-ounce loaf)   1 serving: 1-ounce slice (28 grams)

1 cup cream-style cottage cheese, at room temperature (70° F. or 21° C.)
1 teaspoon salt
1½ tablespoons sugar (needed for yeast action)
2 tablespoons margarine, melted
1 tablespoon dill weed
1 teaspoon grated lemon rind
2 tablespoons finely minced green onions
½ cup lukewarm water (110° F. to 115° F. or 43° C. to 46° C.)
1 package instant active dry yeast
2½ cups flour
2 teaspoons margarine, at room temperature

When cottage cheese is warmed to room temperature, add salt, sugar, melted margarine, dill weed, grated lemon rind, and green onions; mix thoroughly, then set aside. Pour the lukewarm water into a large bowl. Sprinkle yeast on top; stir to dissolve. Stir in cottage cheese mixture; blend thoroughly. Add 1¼ cups flour gradually, beating until smooth. Stir (do not beat) in the remaining 1¼ cups flour gradually, mixing well. Turn onto a lightly floured board; knead until smooth and elastic (about 7 to 8 minutes). Use 1 teaspoon softened margarine to grease a large bowl. Place dough in this bowl and turn it around to lightly grease on all sides. Cover bowl and place in a warm place, free from drafts, until dough doubles in bulk, about 1 hour. (The oven, turned off, works well for this.) Punch down in 4 or 5 places, turn out on a board, and let the dough rest for 15 minutes. Meanwhile, grease a 9-by-5-by-3-inch loaf pan with remaining 1 teaspoon softened margarine. Shape dough into a loaf and place in the prepared pan. Cover; let rise in a warm place until center is slightly higher than edge of pan (about 1 hour). Preheat oven to 400° F. (205° C.) 10 minutes before rising time is up. Bake loaf about 50 minutes.

Nutritive values per serving: CHO 13 gm., PRO 3 gm., FAT 2 gm.,
Calories 85, Sodium 137 mg.

Food Exchange per serving: 1 Bread Exchange plus ½ Fat Exchange.

Low-sodium diets: Omit salt. Use unsalted margarine.

Mustard Whole Wheat Bread

This bread, served with ham or roast beef, is a real treat for picnics.

20 slices (yield: 1¼-pound loaf)   1 serving: 1-ounce slice (28 grams)

2 packages instant active dry yeast
¾ cup lukewarm water (110° F. to 115° F. or 43° C. to 46° C.)
2 teaspoons sugar (Don't worry, it's OK.)
1⅓ cups unsifted white flour
1 teaspoon salt
3 tablespoons margarine, melted
⅓ cup Dijon mustard
1⅓ cups whole wheat flour
2 teaspoons vegetable oil (to oil pans)

Combine yeast, lukewarm water, and sugar in a large bowl; stir until yeast is completely dissolved. Add the white flour gradually, beating until smooth. Cover bowl, set in a warm place, and let rise until surface is all bubbly and batter is light (30 to 40 minutes). Add salt, margarine, and mustard; mix well. Add whole wheat flour gradually, mixing thoroughly. Turn onto a lightly floured board and knead for 10 minutes, or until light and elastic. Place in a large, oiled bowl, turning dough over several times to form a ball that is well coated. Cover bowl and set in a warm place until the dough is doubled in size, about 1 to 2 hours. Punch down in several places, turn onto a lightly floured board, and knead for 5 minutes. Let rest, covered, for 10 minutes. Shape into a loaf and place in an oiled 8½-by-4½-by-2½-inch loaf pan. Cover, let rise until doubled in size. When almost ready, preheat oven to 375° F. (190° C.). Bake 40 to 45 minutes.

Nutritive values per serving: CHO 14 gm., PRO 2 gm., FAT 3 gm., Calories 86, Sodium 212 mg.

Food Exchanges per serving: 1 Bread Exchange plus ½ Fat Exchange.

Low-sodium diets: Omit salt. Use unsalted margarine.

Hotsy Totsy Buns

18 buns   1 serving: 1 bun

¾ cup skim milk
2 tablespoons sugar (needed for yeast action)
1½ teaspoons salt
4 tablespoons margarine
2 packages instant active dry yeast
¾ cup lukewarm water (110° F. to 115° F. or 43° C. to 46° C.)
4½ cups sifted flour
1 egg, beaten
¼ cup prepared mild mustard
¾ cup finely chopped onion
1 tablespoon vegetable oil for bowl and pans

Heat milk in the top of a double boiler until skin begins to form on surface. Stir in sugar, salt, and margarine; mix well, then let stand to cool until lukewarm. Add yeast to lukewarm water in a large bowl; stir until dissolved. Stir in the lukewarm milk mixture; mix well. Gently stir in 1 cup of flour, then the beaten egg, mustard, and onions. Stir in another 1¼ cups flour, beating until smooth. Gradually stir in about another 2¼ cups flour, working it in carefully. Turn onto a lightly floured board and knead until smooth and elastic. Place in a large bowl oiled with 1 teaspoon of the 1 tablespoon of vegetable oil; turn ball of dough around so it will be well oiled. Cover bowl lightly. Let rise in a warm place, free from drafts, about 40 minutes or until doubled in bulk. Punch down and let rest for 10 minutes. Turn out onto a lightly floured board. Shape into eighteen 2½-inch balls and place ½ inch apart on oiled baking sheets. With palm of hand pat down gently to flatten slightly. Preheat oven to 375° F. (190° C.). Cover buns lightly and let rise just until oven is heated. Brush lightly with remaining vegetable oil. Bake about 18 to 20 minutes.

Nutritive values per serving: CHO 25 gm., PRO 4 gm., FAT 4 gm., Calories 154, Sodium 260 mg.

Food Exchanges per serving: 1½ Bread Exchanges plus 1 Fat Exchange. If allowed only 1 Bread Exchange at a meal, use ½ bun.

Low-sodium diets: This recipe is not suitable.

SANDWICHES

Baked Cheese Toastwiches

2 sandwiches   1 serving: 1 sandwich

4 slices bread
1 egg, beaten with fork
2 tablespoons skim milk
¼ teaspoon salt
2 dashes paprika
4 slices (1 ounce each) American cheese

Preheat oven to 400° F. (205° C.). Prepare shallow baking pan with vegetable pan coating (spray or solid). Toast bread on one side only. Combine beaten egg, milk, salt, and paprika; mix well, and pour into a pie plate. Dip bread in this mixture quickly until all is absorbed. Place 2 slices bread toasted side down in prepared pan, cover each with 1 slice cheese. Place remaining 2 slices bread toasted side up on top, then cover with remaining 2 slices cheese. Bake 10 to 12 minutes.

Nutritive values per serving: CHO 30 gm., PRO 21 gm., FAT 21 gm., Calories 404, Sodium 1,230 mg.

Food Exchanges per serving: 2 Bread Exchanges plus 3 Medium-Fat Meat Exchanges plus 1 Fat Exchange.

Low-sodium diets: Omit salt. Use low-sodium bread and low-sodium cheese.

Cheese Sandwich Spread

8 servings (yield: 2 cups)   1 serving: ¼ cup

1 cup cream-style cottage cheese, small curd
1 package (3 ounces) cream cheese
½ cup (2 ounces) finely diced American cheese
1 teaspoon lemon juice
⅛ teaspoon paprika
6 medium pimiento-stuffed olives, finely chopped
¼ cup finely chopped green onion
½ teaspoon Worcestershire sauce

Measure all ingredients into a large mixing bowl. Using an electric mixer, beat at slow speed for 30 seconds, then gradually increase to high speed; beat for 3 minutes. Store in a covered jar in the refrigerator several hours before serving.

Nutritive values per serving: CHO 2 gm., PRO 6 gm., FAT 8 gm.,
Calories 103, Sodium 212 mg.

Food Exchange per serving: 1 High-Fat Meat Exchange.

Low-sodium diets: This recipe is not suitable.

Chicken Salad Baked in Nests

Students at Mundelein College tested this recipe and they judged it a prize winner.

4 servings   1 serving: 1 nest

4 hard rolls (about 50 grams each)
½ cup Lemon Mayonnaise (*see* Index)
1½ teaspoons curry powder
1½ cups lightly packed, diced, cooked chicken
½ cup diced tomato
¼ cup finely cut green onions
2 slices (1 ounce each) American cheese, cut in half

Preheat oven to 350° F. (180° C.). Cut top off rolls and scoop out soft bread from inside. Each remaining "nest" should weigh about

20 grams; discard scooped out portions. Mix Lemon Mayonnaise and curry powder; add chicken, tomatoes, and onions and mix again. Spoon mixture into the nests (each nest will hold ½ cup of the mixture). Place nests in a shallow baking pan and cover with foil. Bake 20 minutes; remove foil and put ½ slice of American cheese on top of each; continue baking, uncovered, 8 to 10 minutes until cheese melts.

Nutritive values per serving: CHO 15 gm., PRO 28 gm., FAT 8 gm., Calories 250, Sodium 606 mg.

Food Exchanges per serving: 1 Bread Exchange plus 4 Lean Meat Exchanges.

Low-sodium diets: Omit salt in Lemon Mayonnaise. Use low-sodium cheese.

Egg Salad Sandwich Filling

2 servings (yield: ⅔ cup) 1 serving: ⅓ cup

2 hard-cooked eggs, peeled and chilled
1 tablespoon finely chopped green onion
1 tablespoon finely chopped celery and leaves
¼ teaspoon salt
Dash of pepper
3 tablespoons Lemon Mayonnaise (*see* Index)
½ teaspoon hot prepared mustard

Finely dice the eggs; mix thoroughly with all other ingredients. Cover and chill for at least 1 hour or until flavors are well blended. Use as a spread for open-face sandwiches or as a sandwich filling. This may also be mounded on crisp lettuce, garnished with a dash of paprika, and served as a salad.

Nutritive values per serving
(filling only): CHO 2 gm., PRO 6 gm., FAT 6 gm., Calories 87, Sodium 547 mg.

Food Exchange per serving
(filling only): 1 Medium-Fat Meat Exchange.

Low-sodium diets: Omit salt in this recipe and in recipe for Lemon Mayonnaise.

Egg and Olive Spread

5 servings (yield: 1¼ cups)   1 serving: ¼ cup

4 hard-cooked eggs, chilled
½ cup pimiento-stuffed olives
2½ tablespoons finely chopped onions
¼ cup Low-Calorie Cooked Dressing (see Index)
¼ teaspoon salt
⅛ teaspoon pepper
¼ teaspoon dry mustard
½ teaspoon prepared horseradish

Shell eggs. Finely chop eggs and olives; add remaining ingredients and mix well. Store in a tightly covered jar in the refrigerator.

Nutritive values per serving
   (spread only):   CHO 2 gm., PRO 5 gm., FAT 6 gm.,
                               Calories 85, Sodium 520 mg.

Food Exchange per serving
   (spread only):   1 Medium-Fat Meat Exchange.

Low-sodium diets: Omit salt. Substitute green or red sweet peppers
                  for the olives. Omit salt and use unsalted marga-
                  rine in the dressing recipe.

Pizza Snacks

3 servings   1 serving: 1 pizza

3 slices fresh bread
2 tablespoons catsup
1 tablespoon finely cut green pepper
1 tablespoon finely cut mushrooms
Dash of oregano or basil
¼ cup shredded mozzarella cheese

Roll bread slices flat and thin with a rolling pin or an empty quart jar. Place on a flat pan 3 inches under the broiler; heat until lightly toasted on one side, then remove from oven. Turn slices over and spread untoasted sides with a layer of each of the remaining ingredients, in the order listed, ending with a sprinkling of cheese. Broil until cheese melts and browns slightly. To serve, cut each pizza in quarters.

Nutritive values per serving: CHO 17 gm., PRO 6 gm., FAT 5 gm., Calories 141, Sodium 317 mg.

Food Exchanges per serving: 1 Bread Exchange plus 1 Medium-Fat Meat Exchange.

Low-sodium diets: Use low-sodium bread and low-sodium catsup.

Tuna and Cheese Broil

These open-face sandwiches are great as a lunch or supper entrée.

4 servings   1 serving: 1 sandwich

1 can (7 ounces) tuna, packed in water
4 tablespoons Lemon Dressing *(see* Index)
2 tablespoons finely cut kosher dill pickle
2 teaspoons prepared mustard
½ teaspoon Worcestershire sauce
4 slices bread, toasted on one side
4 slices tomato
1 cup grated cheese (American, Cheddar, or Colby)

Drain tuna; flake to separate. Combine tuna, Lemon Dressing, pickles, mustard, and Worcestershire sauce; mix well. Spread on untoasted sides of bread. Top with a tomato slice and sprinkle with cheese. Broil just until cheese is bubbly.

Nutritive values per serving: CHO 16 gm., PRO 24 gm., FAT 10 gm., Calories 260, Sodium 748 mg.

Food Exchanges per serving: 1 Bread Exchange plus 3 Lean Meat Exchanges.

Low-sodium diets: This recipe is not suitable.

Tuna Danish

6 servings (yield of tuna mixture: 4 cups)   1 serving: ⅔ cup tuna
                                                    mixture plus 1 slice toast

2 cans (7 ounces each) tuna, packed in oil
1 cup coarsely grated cabbage
⅔ cup grated carrots
½ cup plain, low-fat yogurt
3 tablespoons catsup
1½ tablespoons vinegar
½ teaspoon salt
Few grains of pepper
6 slices bread, toasted
½ head lettuce
18 thin slices pared cucumber
⅛ teaspoon paprika

Drain tuna, then flake lightly. Combine tuna, cabbage, and carrots; set aside. Combine yogurt, catsup, vinegar, salt, and pepper; mix well. Add to tuna mixture and blend. Put 1 piece of toast on each plate; add several lettuce leaves. Add ⅔ cup of tuna mixture. Arrange 3 slices of cucumber across top. Sprinkle lightly with paprika.

Nutritive values per serving: CHO 18 gm., PRO 20 gm., FAT 6 gm., Calories 208, Sodium 750 mg.

Food Exchanges per serving: 1 Bread Exchange plus 2½ Low-Fat Meat Exchanges.

Low-sodium diets: Omit salt. Use unsalted tuna, low-sodium catsup, and low-sodium bread.

Tuna Sandwich Filling

3 servings (yield: ¾ cup)   1 serving: ¼ cup

1 can (3½ ounces) tuna, packed in oil
¼ cup finely cut celery
1 tablespoon finely cut green pepper
⅛ teaspoon salt
Few grains of pepper
1 tablespoon finely cut green onions
¼ cup plain, low-fat yogurt
1 teaspoon lemon juice or vinegar
1 tablespoon grated American cheese

Drain tuna well, then flake it into a bowl. Add all remaining
ingredients and mix well. Use ¼ cup to spread on one slice of bread
for an open-face sandwich or between 2 slices bread for a regular
sandwich.

Nutritive values per serving
  (filling only):   CHO 2 gm., PRO 9 gm., FAT 3
                                           gm., Calories 77, Sodium 321 mg.

Food Exchange per serving
  (filling only):   1 Lean Meat Exchange.

Low-sodium diets: Omit salt. Use unsalted tuna.

Western Sandwich Spread

2 servings (yield: ⅔ cup)   1 serving: ⅓ cup

2 hard-cooked eggs, chilled
2 teaspoons finely chopped green onion
2 tablespoons tomato catsup
½ cup finely chopped cooked ham or 2 pieces
  cooked Canadian-style bacon, finely chopped

Shell eggs; chop or finely grate eggs. Combine eggs with all remaining ingredients and mix well.

Nutritive values per serving
  (spread only):   CHO 4 gm., PRO 15 gm., FAT 8
                                    gm., Calories 154, Sodium 527 mg.

Food Exchanges per serving
  (spread only):   1 Vegetable Exchange plus 2 Lean
                                    Meat Exchanges.

Low-sodium diets: This recipe is not suitable.

28

Meats

BEEF

Roast Beef

Choose a rib, sirloin, rump, or eye of round roast. The rump roast is the least tender of these cuts. Select a compact or tied piece of meat so that it will cook evenly. A boneless roast should be no smaller than 3 pounds because very small roasts become dry and toughen easily. Meat authorities advise that a boned roast yields about 3 servings per pound; roasts with bones yield only 1 to 2 servings per pound depending on the amount of bone and fat.

The roasts listed below are tender cuts and are usually cooked without adding liquid. Season the roast with any combination of seasonings you prefer. Then place the roast, fat side up for natural basting, on a rack in a shallow roasting pan. Insert a meat thermometer into the thickest part of the meat muscle, not touching the bone.

Cook the meat uncovered in a 325° F. (165° C.) oven. When beef is done this will register 140° F. (60° C.) for rare, 150° F. (65° C.) for medium rare, 160° F. (70° C.) for medium, and 170° F. (75° C.) for well-done.

Roasts can be carved more easily if they stand out of the oven about 15 to 20 minutes after cooking. Since they continue to cook during this time, remove beef from the oven 5° below the temperature you desire.

As a general guide for approximate total cooking times, multiply the cooking time per pound by the weight of the roast. These times are based on medium-rare beef:

> Standing rib—25 to 30 minutes per pound.
> Rolled rib—about 35 minutes per pound.
> Rump—20 to 25 minutes per pound.
> Rolled rump—25 to 30 minutes per pound.
> Sirloin—20 to 25 minutes per pound.
> Sirloin tip—about 30 minutes per pound.
> Round—20 to 25 minutes per pound.

Of course, if you want your meat medium or well-done, cooking times will be longer. A meat thermometer is the best method for accuracy. These roasting guidelines and timetables are based on Choice grade of beef. Lesser grade cuts of beef are better for braising or other moist cooking methods.

Nutritive values per serving (3 ounces cooked, boneless meat trimmed of fat; 3 ounces = 2 pieces each 4⅛-by-2¼ inches wide and ¼ inch thick = 85 grams on your scale):

> Rib roast—CHO 0, PRO 24 gm., FAT 16 gm., Calories 250, Sodium 59 mg.
> Round roast—CHO 0, PRO 26 gm., FAT 5 gm., Calories 161, Sodium 65 mg.
> Rump roast—CHO 0, PRO 25 gm., FAT 8 gm., Calories 177, Sodium 61 mg.
> Sirloin roast—CHO 0, PRO 26 gm., FAT 8 gm., Calories 184, Sodium 64 mg.

Food Exchanges per serving (3 ounces):
> Rib roast—3 Medium-Fat Meat Exchanges.
> Round, rump, or sirloin roasts—3 Lean Meat Exchanges.

Low-sodium diets: Do not use salt in seasoning roast.

Roast Beef with Anchovies

12 servings   1 serving: 4 ounces cooked meat

4 pounds eye of round of beef, well trimmed
2 tablespoons olive oil
1 can (2 ounces) flat anchovies, packed in oil
2 teaspoons coarsely ground pepper

Preheat oven to 300° F. (150° C.). Rub beef with olive oil and oil from anchovy can. Cut slits into beef and insert half of the anchovies inside the slits; spread remaining anchovies on top of meat. Sprinkle roast with pepper. Put roast in a shallow roasting pan; cover tightly with foil. For medium rare roast 1 hour. Meat thermometer should read 150° F. (65° C.) for medium rare. Cook longer if you prefer. The estimation of 12 servings is based on a 4-ounce serving each. Nondiabetics can be hearty eaters and may eat more, so plan accordingly.

Nutritive values per serving: CHO 0, PRO 28 gm., FAT 9 gm., Calories 200, Sodium 454 mg.

Food Exchanges per serving: 4 Lean Meat Exchanges.

Low-sodium diets: This recipe is not suitable.

Peppered Rib Eye

Start early because this must be marinated overnight.

About 12 servings (yield: 45 ounces lean meat)

1 serving: 4 ounces lean meat. (Hearty eaters may have larger portions, so plan accordingly.)

6 pounds boneless rib eye roast, well trimmed
⅓ cup peppercorns (more or less to taste)
1 teaspoon ground cardamom
1 cup soy sauce
¾ cup vinegar
1 tablespoon tomato paste
1 teaspoon paprika
½ teaspoon garlic powder

Wipe roast with dampened paper towel. Put peppercorns in a small paper or plastic bag and pound them with a rolling pin or meat mallet until well cracked. Mix cracked pepper and cardamom and press into meat. Mix all remaining ingredients to make a marinade. Pour marinade over meat and store in the refrigerator for 12 hours or longer, turning meat in marinade occasionally. Wrap beef in foil and roast at 300° F. (150° C.) for 2 hours for medium-rare or longer if you prefer.

Nutritive values per serving: CHO 1 gm., PRO 30 gm., FAT 14 gm., Calories 263, Sodium 664 mg.

Food Exchanges per serving: 4 Medium-Fat Meat Exchanges.

Low-sodium diets: This recipe is not suitable.

Roast Beef with Caraway Seeds

7 servings (yield: 1¾ pounds cooked
     before final trimming;
     22 ounces edible lean meat.)

1 serving: 3-ounce
slice of lean beef

¾ cup chopped onion
1 teaspoon salt
1 tablespoon caraway seeds
2½ pounds rolled rump or chuck roast, boneless
1 tablespoon vegetable oil
⅓ cup vinegar
1 cup apple juice, unsweetened
Water

Preheat oven to 325° F. (165° C.). Combine ¼ cup of the onions with salt and caraway seeds. Press this mixture into the roast. In a roasting pan heat the oil and add remaining onions; stir over medium heat for 5 minutes until onions are translucent. Put roast in pan; add vinegar, apple juice, and enough water to cover the bottom of the pan with ½-inch liquid. Bake uncovered about 1½ hours for medium rare, or longer if you prefer. Baste with liquid several times during cooking. Trim away extra fat and discard drippings.

Nutritive values per serving: CHO 2 gm., PRO 26 gm., FAT 10 gm., Calories 209, Sodium 370 mg.

Food Exchanges per serving: 3½ Lean Meat Exchanges.

Low-sodium diets: Substitute 2 cloves garlic, crushed, for the salt.

Party Beef Tenderloin

A whole beef tenderloin, when trimmed, will be approximately 4 pounds (raw).

Have your meat cutter trim a whole or half tenderloin. He will lard it or put strips of fat across the top because it is a very lean cut.

Preheat oven to 450° F. (230° C.). Season roast with garlic and cracked pepper or your favorite seasonings. Put tenderloin on a rack in an uncovered roasting pan and roast 45 to 50 minutes for rare to medium-rare beef. A meat thermometer will register 140° F. (60° C.) for rare meat. This cut is also wonderful cooked on a barbecue but be careful not to overcook it. The diabetic should discard fat from around outside edges of meat. The diabetic's portion should be weighed as cooked lean meat; the number of ounces are approximately equal to the number of allowed Meat Exchanges for that meal.

Nutritive value per serving
   (3 ounces):   CHO 0, PRO 26 gm., FAT 9 gm., Calories 192, Sodium 64 mg.

Food Exchanges per serving
   (3 ounces):   3½ Lean Meat Exchanges.

Low-sodium diets: Do not season meat with salt or other seasonings high in sodium.

Flank Steak Swiss Style

Unless you are able to get prime quality (top, fancy grade) flank steak, do not attempt to just broil it for it will be tough. The best method to cook this very lean cut is by braising, and here is a simple, delicious recipe which follows the basic braising directions of professional meat experts.

6 servings

1 serving: ⅙ of meat plus ⅓ cup gravy and vegetables

1½ pounds flank steak
2 tablespoons flour
1 teaspoon salt
¼ teaspoon coarsely ground black pepper
1 teaspoon dry mustard
2 tablespoons vegetable oil
2 cups hot water
2 beef bouillon cubes
½ cup chopped onion
½ cup chopped celery
¼ cup catsup

Preheat oven to 325°F. (165°C.). Cut meat into 6 equal individual serving pieces. Combine flour, salt, pepper, and mustard; mix well and place in a paper bag. Shake each piece of meat in the bag to coat evenly with seasoned flour; place floured pieces aside. Heat vegetable oil in a large frying pan over medium heat. Brown meat pieces in hot oil, turning frequently. Place browned meat in a large, shallow casserole; set aside. Put hot water, bouillon cubes, vegetables, and catsup into the frying pan. Stir over medium heat until bouillon cubes are dissolved. Spread vegetable mixture evenly on top of meat. Cover and cook in oven for 2½ hours or until meat is fork tender. Or prepare this recipe on top of the stove in a 12-inch frying pan. After browning meat, spread vegetables on top, combine remaining ingredients until bouillon cubes are dissolved, pour on top of meat, cover pan tightly, and simmer gently 2 to 2½ hours.

Nutritive values per serving: CHO 7 gm., PRO 24 gm., FAT 10 gm., Calories 220, Sodium 848 mg.

Food Exchanges per serving: 3½ Lean Meat Exchanges plus 1 Vegetable Exchange.

Low-sodium diets: Omit salt. Use low-sodium catsup and low-sodium beef bouillon cubes.

Berna's Round Steak

6 servings (yield: 4 cups)   1 serving: ⅔ cup

2 pounds round steak
2 tablespoons vegetable oil
½ teaspoon ginger
¼ teaspoon garlic powder
½ teaspoon salt
2 cups beef bouillon
1 tablespoon cornstarch
2 tablespoons water
1 tablespoon soy sauce
1 green pepper, cut into thin strips

Cut off separable fat and discard. Cut lean meat into ½-by-3-inch strips. Brown meat in oil. Add ginger, garlic powder, salt, and bouillon. Bring to a boil, lower heat, and cover pan. Cook for 1 hour or until tender. Blend cornstarch, water, and soy sauce and stir this mixture into the pan. Add green pepper and cook a few minutes until sauce is thickened and clear.

Nutritive values per serving: CHO 2 gm., PRO 29 gm., FAT 10 gm., Calories 220, Sodium 790 mg.

Food Exchanges per serving: 4 Lean Meat Exchanges.

Low-sodium diets: Omit salt. Use low-sodium bouillon. Substitute low-sodium Worcestershire sauce for soy sauce.

Creole Steak

7 servings

1 serving: 3 ounces meat
plus ½ cup rice mixture

2 pounds lean round steak
¼ cup flour
2 teaspoons salt
2 teaspoons paprika
½ teaspoon pepper
3 tablespoons vegetable oil
1 cup chopped onions
⅓ cup chopped green peppers
1 can (16 ounces) tomatoes
½ cup raw rice
1 cup condensed beef broth
1 cup water

Cut steak into 7 equal serving pieces. Mix flour, salt, paprika, and pepper; dredge meat in mixture. Heat oil in a large frying pan. Lightly brown onions and peppers and remove from oil. Brown meat in remaining oil. Cover meat with onions and green peppers. Cut up tomatoes and add with their liquid to meat. Sprinkle rice into pan; add broth and water. Mix thoroughly. Bring to a boil, turn heat down, and cover tightly. Simmer 1½ hours or until meat is tender, stirring occasionally.

Nutritive values per serving: CHO 21 gm., PRO 30 gm., FAT 22 gm., Calories 409, Sodium 1018 mg.

Food Exchanges per serving: 4 Medium-Fat Meat Exchanges plus 1 Bread Exchange plus 1 Vegetable Exchange.

Low-sodium diets: Omit salt. Use unsalted canned tomatoes and low-sodium beef broth.

Swiss Steak

6 servings   1 serving: 4 ounces steak plus ½ cup sauce

1 (2 pounds) round steak, ¾ inch thick
2 tablespoons flour
1 teaspoon salt
½ teaspoon pepper
1 tablespoon vegetable oil
1 can (16 ounces) tomatoes, cut up, with liquid
1 cup chopped onions
1 medium green pepper, sliced
1 can (2½ ounces) sliced mushrooms
1 tablespoon cornstarch
¼ cup cold water

Trim fat and bone from meat and divide meat into 6 portions. Mix flour, salt, and ¼ teaspoon pepper together and sprinkle over both sides of meat; pound flour mixture into meat with a meat mallet or the side of a heavy plate. Brown meat in vegetable oil in a heavy frying pan. Add tomatoes, tomato liquid, and onions; cover and bring to boil. Reduce heat and simmer about 2 hours or until meat is tender. Add green peppers and mushrooms during last 10 minutes of cooking. Put meat on heated platter leaving tomato mixture in frying pan. Blend cornstarch into cold water; blend into pan liquids and add remaining ¼ teaspoon pepper. Cook, stirring constantly, until gravy is thickened.

Nutritive values per serving: CHO 10 gm., PRO 32 gm., FAT 21 gm., Calories 364, Sodium 567 mg.

Food Exchanges per serving: 4 Medium-Fat Meat Exchanges plus 2 Vegetable Exchanges.

Low-sodium diets: Omit salt. Use unsalted canned tomatoes.

Joan's Beef Oriental

4 servings (yield: 4 cups)   1 serving: 1 cup

1 pound lean round steak, ¼ inch thick
2 tablespoons vegetable oil
1½ cups hot water
1 beef bouillon cube
1 tablespoon soy sauce
1 clove garlic, crushed
⅛ teaspoon coarsely ground black pepper
½ cup (56 grams) raw carrot strips (3 by ¼ inches)
½ cup slant-sliced celery
1 cup firmly packed, slant-sliced green onions
1 cup sweet green peppers, cut into 1-inch squares
2½ cups (about ½ pound) sliced, fresh mushrooms
½ cup drained, sliced water chestnuts
1 to 1½ cups boiling water
2 tablespoons cornstarch
¼ cup cold water

If time allows, partially freeze meat for easier slicing. Remove and discard fat around outside; cut meat into thin strips, 3 to 4 inches long and ⅛ inch thick. Heat oil in a large, heavy frying pan. Brown meat strips, stirring with a wooden spoon to brown all over. Add 1½ cups hot water, beef bouillon cube, soy sauce, garlic, and black pepper. Cover and simmer very slowly for 40 minutes. Meanwhile, prepare vegetables. When meat is cooked, add vegetables in order listed, spreading evenly. If meat is cooked almost dry add 1½ cups boiling water; otherwise, add 1 cup. Cover, and let cook over low heat 10 minutes. Mix cornstarch into cold water. Add slowly to liquid in pot. Stir and cook over moderate heat until thick, smooth, and clear.

Nutritive values per serving: CHO 14 gm., PRO 26 gm., FAT 18 gm., Calories 320, Sodium 450 mg.

Food Exchanges per serving: 3 Medium-Fat Meat Exchanges plus 2 Vegetable Exchanges.

Low-sodium diets: Use low-sodium bouillon cube. Substitute low-sodium Worcestershire sauce for soy sauce.

Japanese Steak and Pea Pods

If the steak is partially frozen it will be much easier to slice. After cutting, thaw to room temperature before cooking. This is a stir-fry recipe.

4 servings (yield: 4 cups)   1 serving: 1 cup

1½ pounds sirloin with fat and bone
2 tablespoons soy sauce
2 tablespoons dry sherry
1 tablespoon vegetable oil
1 cup slant-sliced celery
¾ cup slant-sliced green onions, with tops
1 package (6 ounces) frozen Chinese pea pods, thawed
¾ cup tomato juice

Remove from meat all fat and bone and discard. Cut meat into strips 1-by-2-by-½-inch. Mix the soy sauce and sherry together and pour over the steak strips; allow to marinate 10 minutes. Meanwhile prepare the vegetables. Heat oil in a 10- or 12-inch frying pan over high heat. Brown the meat quickly while stirring vigorously. Add the celery and onions; cover, lower heat to medium, and cook 3 minutes. Add pea pods and tomato juice, and cook, stirring, until pea pods are hot but still crisp. The total cooking time is only about 7 or 8 minutes.

Nutritive values per serving: CHO 11 gm., PRO 39 gm., FAT 13 gm., Calories 331, Sodium 887 mg.

Food Exchanges per serving: 5 Lean Meat Exchanges plus 2 Vegetable Exchanges.

Low-sodium diets.   Substitute low-sodium Worcestershire sauce for the soy sauce and use unsalted tomato juice

Hotcha Baked Beef

4 servings   1 serving: 1 piece meat plus 2 tablespoons sauce

1 pound lean boneless round steak, ¾ inch thick
1 tablespoon vegetable oil
½ cup finely cut onions
1 cup Hotcha Beef Sauce (*see* Index)
4 rings sweet green pepper

Preheat oven to 300° F. (150° C.). Cut steak into 4 serving pieces. Heat oil in a frying pan, turn heat to medium, and cook onions until lightly browned, stirring frequently; push to one side of pan. Brown meat pieces on both sides, turning twice. Transfer meat and onions to a large, shallow casserole. Pour Hotcha Beef Sauce in frying pan, bring to a boil, and pour evenly over meat in the casserole. Cover and bake 2 hours, basting occasionally. Five minutes before dish is done, remove cover and place 1 green pepper ring on top of each serving; finish cooking.

Nutritive values per serving: CHO 10 gm., PRO 25 gm., FAT 18 gm., Calories 297, Sodium 746 mg.

Food Exchanges per serving: 3½ Medium-Fat Meat Exchanges plus 1 Fruit Exchange.

Low-sodium diets: Modify Hotcha Beef Sauce as directed in that recipe.

Old-Fashioned Beef Stew

This recipe may be simmered in a large covered pot on top of the stove. The oven method saves pot watching. If you prefer Old-Fashioned Lamb Stew, choose lean lamb and add 1 teaspoon extra dill.

4 servings (yield: 4 cups)   1 serving: 1 cup

¼ cup flour
1¼ teaspoons salt
⅛ teaspoon black pepper
¼ teaspoon dry mustard
1¼ pounds top round steak, 1 inch thick
1 tablespoon vegetable oil
2½ cups water
1 teaspoon Worcestershire sauce
2 cups pared, quartered, and sliced potatoes (about 13 ounces)
1 cup sliced onions
1 cup carrots, sliced crosswise
½ teaspoon dill weed (optional)

Preheat oven to 350°F. (180°C.). Combine flour, salt, pepper, and mustard in a paper bag. Trim off all fat around outside of round steak; cut meat into 1-inch cubes. Shake meat cubes in the paper bag with flour, a few at a time, until well coated. Heat oil in a large frying pan; brown meat cubes over medium heat, turning with tongs until meat is evenly browned. Transfer meat cubes to a 2½-quart casserole; set aside. Sprinkle seasoned flour remaining in paper bag into the fat remaining in the frying pan; stir vigorously until smooth and mixed. Add water very slowly and stir; add Worcestershire sauce. Cook and stir until smooth; pour on top of meat in casserole. Cover and cook in the oven for 2 hours. Mix vegetables and dill weed into meat, cover, and cook in oven for 1 more hour or until meat and vegetables are tender.

Nutritive values per serving: CHO 25 gm., PRO 26 gm., FAT 18 gm., Calories 365, Sodium 816 mg.

Food Exchanges per serving: 1 Bread Exchange plus 2 Vegetable Exchanges plus 3 Medium-Fat Meat Exchanges.

Low-sodium diets: Omit salt. Use low-sodium Worcestershire sauce.

GROUND BEEF

Ground beef may be purchased in bulk, loaves, or patties. Ground round steak is supposed to be leaner than meat labeled "ground chuck," "ground beef," or "hamburger." Meat labeled "ground round" is often more expensive because it contains more lean meat and less fat. But most meat cutters do not separate and weigh the lean versus the fat portions, although meat labeled 80% or 85% lean would suggest this care.

Diabetics should select the leanest possible ground beef. We recommend that you choose a piece of lean round steak, and ask the meat cutter to grind the meat once for you. Twice ground makes it too fine and solid. If the piece of round steak you select has a wide band of fat around the outside, have the piece trimmed before it is ground.

Recipes in this book using ground beef are calculated on the basis of the beef being 85% lean, ground round.

Ground meat, like organ meats, is highly perishable and cannot be stored at refrigerator temperatures (35° F. to 40° F.) for more than 2 days. If longer storage is necessary, wrap meat and freeze it until desired for use.

Kay's Favorite Meat Loaf

This meat loaf is great cold, served plain or in sandwiches. Good hot, too!

6 to 8 servings

1 serving: 1 large slice (4½-by-2-by-1-inch; 140 grams) *or* 1 medium slice (4½-by-2-by-¾-inch; 105 grams)

1 beef bouillon cube
½ cup boiling water
2 slices bread, finely crumbled
1½ pounds 85% lean ground beef
2 medium eggs, beaten slightly
½ cup finely chopped onion
¼ cup finely chopped celery
2 teaspoons Worcestershire sauce
1 tablespoon catsup

Preheat oven to 350°F. (180°C.). Line a square, shallow (8-by-8-inch) baking pan with foil. Dissolve beef bouillon cube in boiling water in a large bowl. Add all other ingredients except the catsup and blend well with a fork. Turn onto foil in pan and, with hands, shape quickly into a 6-by-4½-by-2-inch loaf. With the dull edge of a knife make a crisscross pattern across the top; spread catsup on top. Cover loaf with a tent of foil that does not touch the top. Bake for 45 minutes. Remove foil; bake uncovered for another 45 minutes. Remove from oven and cool in pan for 2 to 3 minutes before serving. Using this molded method instead of a loaf pan allows the fat to drain from the loaf, whereas a loaf pan retains fat.

Nutritive values per serving:
1 large slice—   CHO 7 gm., PRO 26 gm., FAT 16 gm., Calories 290, Sodium 386 mg.
1 medium slice—   CHO 5 gm., PRO 20 gm., FAT 12 gm., Calories 216, Sodium 287 mg.

Food Exchanges per serving:
1 large slice—   3½ Medium-Fat Meat Exchanges plus ½ Bread Exchange.
1 medium slice—   3 Medium-Fat Meat Exchanges plus 1 Vegetable Exchange.

Low-sodium diets: Omit salt. Use low-sodium bouillon cube, low-sodium Worcestershire sauce, and low-sodium catsup.

Ground Beef Patties

Americans consumed one billion hamburgers last year! This is an excellent basic recipe with two delicious variations.

4 to 6 servings   1 serving: 1 large *or* 1 small patty

1 pound 85% lean beef, ground once
1 teaspoon salt
½ teaspoon dry mustard
¼ teaspoon pepper
1 tablespoon water
2 teaspoons Worcestershire sauce

Combine seasonings and liquid, sprinkle on top of meat, and mix well together. To make 4 meat patties, measure ½ cup for each. To make 6 meat patties, measure ⅓ cup for each. Shape lightly into patties.

To *oven broil* remove broiler rack from oven; preheat broiler for 10 minutes. Arrange patties on cold rack and place rack 3 inches below broiler heat. For thick patties broil 4 to 6 minutes on each side, turning once with a wide spatula. Thin patties will require 3 to 5 minutes on each side.

To *pan broil* use a Teflon frying pan or a heavy, regular metal frying pan prepared with vegetable pan coating (spray or solid). Heat pan over high heat for about 30 seconds. Add meat patties and brown meat patties on both sides, then turn heat to medium and cook 4 to 8 minutes. Do not press down on patties with spatula or "spank" them, or you will get dry patties.

Nutritive values per serving:
    1 large patty—   CHO 0, PRO 23 gm., FAT 14 gm., Calories 230, Sodium 690 mg.
    1 small patty—   CHO 0, PRO 16 gm., FAT 10 gm., Calories 153, Sodium 460 mg.

Food Exchanges per serving:
    1 large patty—   3 Medium-Fat Meat Exchanges.
    1 small patty—   2 Medium-Fat Meat Exchanges.

Low-sodium diets: Omit salt. Use low-sodium Worcestershire sauce.

Cheeseburgers

After turning meat patties once, place on top of each patty a 1-ounce slice of American cheese. Finish cooking. This will add 1 High-Fat Meat Exchange to values of each patty (CHO 0, PRO 6 gm., FAT 9 gm., Calories 106, Sodium 406 mg.).

Baked Barbecued Patties

After browning meat patties on both sides transfer them to a shallow casserole. Spread 1 tablespoon of Barbecue Sauce (*see* Index) over each patty. Cover casserole. Bake in a 350°F. (180°C.) oven for 15 minutes. Up to 1 tablespoon sauce for 1 serving is "free." Follow directions in Barbecue Sauce recipe for low-sodium diets.

Beef Porcupines in Tomato Gravy

4 servings (yield: 20 meatballs plus 1⅓ cups gravy)

1 serving: 5 meatballs plus ⅓ cup gravy

1 pound 85% lean ground beef
¼ cup (46 grams) long-grain rice
¼ cup dry bread crumbs
1 teaspoon salt
2 tablespoons minced parsley
2 tablespoons water
1 tablespoon vegetable oil
1 can (10½ ounces) tomato soup
½ teaspoon garlic powder
1 teaspoon Worcestershire sauce
2 cups water

Combine ground beef, rice, bread crumbs, salt, parsley, and 2 tablespoons water. Shape into an 8-inch square or pack evenly in an 8-inch square pan. Cut 3 lines on one side and 4 lines on the other side to make 20 equal sections; shape each section into a meatball. Heat oil in a large skillet; brown meatballs in hot oil over medium heat, turning frequently. Combine tomato soup, garlic powder, Worcestershire sauce, and 2 cups water. Add to meatballs; cover and simmer gently for 1 hour or until rice is tender. Serve meatballs with tomato gravy from pan.

Nutritive values per serving: CHO 24 gm., PRO 26 gm., FAT 20 gm., Calories 381, Sodium 1290 mg.

Food Exchanges per serving: 1½ Bread Exchanges plus 3 Medium-Fat Meat Exchanges plus 1 Fat Exchange.

Low-sodium diets: Omit salt. Use unsalted tomato soup and low-sodium Worcestershire sauce.

Beef Crust Pizza

6 servings (yield: a 10-inch pizza)   1 serving: ⅙ of pizza

CRUST
1 pound 85% lean ground beef
1 slice bread, finely crumbled
1 medium egg, beaten
2 teaspoons onion powder
½ teaspoon garlic powder
1 teaspoon salt
¼ teaspoon pepper
½ teaspoon oregano

FILLING
1 can (6 ounces) tomato paste
½ teaspoon basil
1¼ cups thinly sliced sweet green pepper
1 can (4 ounces) mushroom pieces, drained
4 ounces shredded mozzarella cheese

Preheat oven to 375° F. (190° C.). Combine all crust ingredients and mix thoroughly. Press into a 10-inch pie pan to form a crust. Bake 10 minutes. Leaving crust in the pie pan, drain off all liquid fat. Spread tomato paste on bottom and sides of crust, then sprinkle with basil. Spread even layers of sliced green peppers, mushrooms, and cheese. Bake 15 minutes. Serve immediately, cutting pizza into six equal wedges.

Nutritive values per serving: CHO 10 gm., PRO 22 gm., FAT 13 gm., Calories 246, Sodium 739 mg.

Food Exchanges per serving: 2½ Medium-Fat Meat Exchanges plus 2 Vegetable Exchanges.

Low-sodium diets: Omit salt. Use unsalted tomato paste and unsalted canned mushrooms.

Meat and Vegetable Casserole

5 servings (yield: 5 cups)   1 serving: 1 cup

1 pound 85% lean ground beef
1 teaspoon salt
½ teaspoon chili powder
⅛ teaspoon allspice
⅛ teaspoon black pepper
1 cup pared, sliced raw potatoes
1 cup chopped onions
1½ cups finely cut celery and leaves
1 can (16 ounces) tomatoes
½ teaspoon vegetable oil (to oil casserole)
½ cup beef broth
¼ cup shredded American cheese

Preheat oven to 350° F. (180° C.). Partially cook meat in a large frying pan over moderate heat; sprinkle with salt, chili powder, allspice, and pepper; continue cooking, stirring frequently with a kitchen fork. When meat has changed color all over, remove pan from heat. Meanwhile, prepare vegetables; cut tomatoes in bite-sized pieces but do not drain. Place alternate layers of meat and vegetables in a lightly oiled 1½- to 2-quart casserole. Pour beef broth on top. Scatter cheese over surface. Cover and bake about 2 hours; uncover the last 10 minutes of cooking.

Nutritive values per serving:	CHO 14 gm., PRO 23 gm., FAT 14 gm., Calories 273, Sodium 799 mg.
Food Exchanges per serving:	1 Bread Exchange plus 3 Medium-Fat Meat Exchanges
Low-sodium diets:	Omit salt. Substitute unsalted canned tomatoes and low-sodium broth. Use low-sodium cheese.

Beef and Zucchini Casserole

6 servings (yield: 6 cups)   1 serving: 1 cup

2 teaspoons vegetable oil
½ cup finely cut onions
1 pound (3 small) zucchini
1 can (4 ounces) mushroom pieces
1 pound 85% lean ground beef
1 can (16 ounces) tomatoes
¼ teaspoon salt
½ teaspoon garlic powder
½ teaspoon oregano
¼ cup grated Parmesan cheese

Preheat oven to 350° F. (180° C.). Heat oil in a frying pan; add onions and stir over medium heat until onions are tender and light golden in color. Wash zucchini, discard ends, and cut crosswise in ¼-inch slices; add to onions; add mushrooms and liquid in can; cook and stir for 3 to 4 minutes over medium heat. Turn into a 2-quart casserole. Turn ground beef into the frying pan, stir over medium heat, and cook until color changes; drain well. Cut up canned tomatoes in their own liquid; add salt, garlic powder, and oregano to tomatoes. Add to meat and mix well. Add meat mixture to zucchini in casserole. Mix carefully. Sprinkle cheese on top. Bake 35 to 40 minutes.

Nutritive values per serving: CHO 8 gm., PRO 19 gm., FAT 13 gm., Calories 286, Sodium 231 mg.

Food Exchanges per serving: 3 Medium-Fat Meat Exchanges plus 1 Vegetable Exchange.

Low-sodium diets: Omit salt. Use unsalted canned mushrooms and unsalted canned tomatoes.

Chili Con Carne

6 servings (yield: 4½ cups)   1 serving: ¾ cup

1 pound 85% lean ground beef
1¼ teaspoons salt
1 cup chopped onions
1 cup finely cut celery
½ cup finely cut sweet green pepper
1 can (16 ounces) tomatoes, cut up, with liquid
¼ teaspoon garlic powder
½ teaspoon oregano
1 tablespoon chili powder (more if desired)
1 can (16 ounces) kidney beans
½ cup beef broth

Use a 2½-quart cooking pot, Teflon-lined or prepared with vegetable pan coating (spray or solid). Turn beef into pot, sprinkle with salt; stir over medium heat with a blending fork (not a spoon) until all meat changes color. Add onions, celery, and green pepper; mix well. Cover and cook over medium heat 2 to 3 minutes. Add tomatoes and liquid and all seasonings, mixing well. Bring to a boil; cover, turn heat low, and simmer gently for 25 minutes, stirring occasionally. Add kidney beans and beef broth. Continue cooking over low heat 15 to 20 minutes.

Nutritive values per serving: CHO 20 gm., PRO 22 gm., FAT 9 gm., Calories 242, Sodium 710 mg. If you break crackers on top of chili, count 5 saltines or ½ cup oyster crackers as 68 more calories and add CHO 15 gm., PRO 2 gm.

Food Exchanges per serving: 3 Lean Meat Exchanges plus 1 Bread Exchange plus 1 Vegetable Exchange. If you break crackers on top of chili, count 5 saltines or ½ cup oyster crackers as 1 additional Bread Exchange.

Low-sodium diets: Omit salt. Use unsalted canned tomatoes and low-sodium beef broth. Omit salted crackers. Use unsalted crackers for topping.

Meat-Stuffed Eggplant

4 servings   1 serving: ½ eggplant

2 eggplants (about 1 pound each)
1½ teaspoons salt
¼ teaspoon pepper
1 pound 85% lean ground beef
1 cup chopped onions
1 tablespoon minced parsley
½ teaspoon oregano
1 can (6 ounces) tomato paste
2 tablespoons Worcestershire sauce
1 tablespoon grated Parmesan cheese

Preheat oven to 350° F. (180° C.). Cut eggplants in half lengthwise; scoop out centers leaving ½-inch walls. Sprinkle shells with salt and pepper and place cut side up in a large shallow baking dish. Chop scooped out eggplant centers and set aside. In a large frying pan, brown the meat, stirring; pour off fat. Stir in chopped eggplant, onions, parsley, and oregano. Cook over medium heat about 10 minutes or until tender, stirring occasionally. Add tomato paste and Worcestershire sauce; mix well. Spoon about ¾ cup of the mixture into each eggplant shell. Sprinkle with cheese. Cover with foil and bake 45 to 50 minutes.

Nutritive values per serving: CHO 22 gm., PRO 28 gm., FAT 13 gm., Calories 314, Sodium 949 mg.

Food Exchanges per serving: 3½ Medium-Fat Meat Exchanges plus 1 Bread Exchange plus 1 Vegetable Exchange.

Low-sodium diets·   Omit salt. Use low-sodium Worcestershire sauce and unsalted tomato paste.

Spicy Meatballs with Tomato Sauce

4 servings (yield: 12 meatballs   1 serving: 3 meatballs
        plus 2 cups sauce)   plus ½ cup sauce

1 pound 85% lean ground beef
1 large egg, beaten
¼ cup beef broth
¼ teaspoon dry mustard
1 teaspoon chili powder
½ teaspoon crushed, dried marjoram
⅛ teaspoon garlic powder
½ teaspoon salt
1 slice fresh bread, finely crumbled
1 can (15 ounces) tomato sauce with tomato bits
¼ cup water

Preheat oven to 400° F. (205° C.). Prepare a shallow baking pan
with vegetable pan coating (spray or solid); set aside. Combine all
ingredients except can of tomato sauce and water. Mix meat
ingredients well. Form into 12 balls, allowing 3 level tablespoonfuls
(total 45 grams) for each ball; place in the pan about 2 inches apart.
Bake 18 to 20 minutes. Heat tomato sauce with tomato bits and
water in saucepan. Pour sauce over meatballs prior to serving.

Nutritive values per serving: CHO 11 gm., PRO 27 gm., FAT 16
                                   gm., Calories 295, Sodium 939 mg.

Food Exchanges per serving: 3 Medium-Fat Meat Exchanges plus
                                   2 Vegetable Exchanges.

Low-sodium diets: Omit salt. Substitute water for beef broth. Use
                       low-sodium bread. Substitute low-sodium cat-
                       sup for tomato sauce.

Sloppy Joes

This is one of Kay's most famous recipes. Nondiabetic families with children make this frequently because they like it so much.

6 servings (yield: 3 cups)   1 serving: ½ cup

1 pound lean beef, ground twice
1 teaspoon salt
¼ cup finely chopped onions
¾ cup finely cut celery stalks with leaves
¼ cup chopped sweet green pepper
½ teaspoon grated lemon rind
¼ cup tomato catsup
¾ cup beef broth
½ teaspoon dry mustard
1 teaspoon Worcestershire sauce

Add salt to meat. Turn into a large, dry, cold frying pan. Stir over medium heat with a large kitchen fork (not a spoon) until meat changes color all over, pouring off any liquid fat as it collects. Add onions, celery, and green pepper. Stir and cook 1 to 2 minutes. Combine all remaining ingredients; add to meat and mix well. Bring to a boil, cover; turn heat low and let simmer gently for 15 to 20 minutes, stirring frequently, until cooked and well mixed.

Nutritive values per serving: CHO 5 gm., PRO 17 gm., FAT 8 gm., Calories 161, Sodium 663 mg. When served on 1 slice of bread or ½ hamburger bun, add CHO 15 gm., PRO 2 gm., Calories 68.

Food Exchanges per serving: 2 Medium-Fat Meat Exchanges plus 1 Vegetable Exchange. When served on 1 slice of bread or ½ hamburger bun, add 1 Bread Exchange.

Low-sodium diets: Omit salt. Use low-sodium catsup, low-sodium beef broth, and low-sodium Worcestershire sauce.

Lean Beef Gravy

4 servings (yield: 1 cup)   1 serving: ¼ cup

2 beef bouillon cubes
1 cup boiling water
1 tablespoon finely minced onion
1 tablespoon cornstarch
¼ cup cold water
⅛ teaspoon salt
2 dashes pepper

In a small saucepan, combine bouillon cubes, boiling water, and onions. Simmer gently 2 to 3 minutes, stirring occasionally to dissolve bouillon cubes. Meanwhile combine cornstarch and cold water, stirring with a fork until smooth and well blended. Add gradually to boiling bouillon, stirring constantly. Cook and stir over medium heat until thick, smooth, and transparent. Stir in salt and pepper. May be seasoned with additional desired herbs.

Nutritive values per serving: CHO 2 gm., PRO 0, FAT 0, Calories 11, Sodium 547 mg.

Food Exchanges per serving: Up to ¼ cup may be considered "free."

Low-sodium diets: Omit salt. Use low-sodium bouillon cubes. Add additional herbs or spices (compatible with meat served) to flavor gravy.

Calves Liver and Onions

4 servings   1 serving: 3½ ounces liver plus ¼ cup onions

4 tablespoons flour
1 teaspoon salt
½ teaspoon pepper
1 pound calves liver, sliced ⅜ inch thick (6 to 8 slices)
3 tablespoons margarine
1⅓ cups (220 grams) sliced onions

Mix together flour, salt, and pepper and dredge the liver in the flour mixture.* Heat 2 tablespoons of the margarine in a large frying pan

* Only ½ of the flour mixture will be used to dredge liver and the recipe is calculated on this basis. Discard the rest.

and sauté the onions until they begin to brown. Remove onions from pan; add remaining tablespoon of margarine to the pan and saute the liver 2 to 3 minutes on each side, turning twice with tongs. Add onions and mix with liver. Cook 2 minutes more. Serve immediately.

Nutritive values per serving: CHO 13 gm., PRO 23 gm., FAT 14 gm., Calories 273, Sodium 460 mg.

Food Exchanges per serving: 3 Medium-Fat Meat Exchanges plus 1 Bread Exchange.

Low-sodium diets: Omit salt and use unsalted margarine.

VEAL

Roast Veal

Select very light-colored veal, which is younger and will be more tender. The best cuts for roasting include veal shoulder or rump roasts. Both may be purchased boned and tied if you prefer.

Because veal has very little fat, it is desirable to place 6 to 8 strips of bacon over the roast after adding salt and pepper or whatever seasonings you prefer. Insert a meat thermometer into the thickest part of the meat, not touching the bone. Roast the meat uncovered in a 325° F. (165° C.) oven.

It takes 25 to 35 minutes cooking time per pound of veal or 40 to 45 minutes per pound for boneless rolled veal roasts. When cooked, the meat thermometer will register 170° F. (75° C.), which is well-done.

Nutritive values per serving
(3-ounce roast veal plus ½
strip bacon):   CHO 0, PRO 24 gm., FAT 11 gm., Calories 206, Sodium 360 mg.

Food Exchanges per serving: 3½ Lean Meat Exchanges.

Low-sodium diets: Omit salt from seasoning roast. The bacon may be used because it only contributes 38 mg. sodium per serving.

Baked Veal Chops

4 servings   1 serving: 1 chop

4 lean loin or shoulder veal chops (about 1½ pounds)
⅓ cup skim milk
1 teaspoon salt
¼ teaspoon pepper
Dash of hot pepper sauce
½ cup crushed cornflakes
2 teaspoons basil
1 tablespoon vegetable oil
1 tablespoon lemon juice
1 teaspoon chopped parsley

Soak veal chops in a mixture of milk, salt, pepper, and hot pepper sauce for 30 minutes. Mix cornflakes and basil. Lift chops from milk mixture and dip in cornflake crumbs to coat all over; place on a plate and chill in refrigerator for 1 hour. Preheat oven to 375° F. (190° C.). Use 1 teaspoon of the vegetable oil to coat inside of a shallow baking pan. Place chops in this, then drizzle remaining oil on top. Bake 1 hour or until tender. Drizzle lemon juice and sprinkle parsley on top during last 5 minutes of cooking.

Nutritive values per serving: CHO 9 gm., PRO 28 gm., FAT 19 gm., Calories 308, Sodium 335 mg.

Food Exchanges per serving: 4 Medium-Fat Meat Exchanges plus ½ Bread Exchange.

Low-sodium diets: Omit salt. Use low-sodium cornflakes or low-sodium bread crumbs for the cornflakes.

Veal Piccata

Veal scallops, which are used in this recipe of Mary's, are very thin slices of veal from the round or loin. They should have no visible fat or tendon, and are sometimes cut and sold frozen.

4 servings

1 serving: 3½ ounces cooked veal plus 2 tablespoons lemon sauce

2 tablespoons flour
½ teaspoon salt
¼ teaspoon pepper
1¼ pounds veal scallops, very thinly sliced
3 tablespoons margarine
1 lemon with rind, very thinly sliced, crosswise
⅓ cup dry white wine
⅓ cup lemon juice
2 tablespoons chopped fresh parsley

Combine the flour, salt, and pepper; sprinkle on both sides of veal scallops. Heat half of the margarine over medium heat in a very large frying pan and quickly sauté half of the veal 2 to 3 minutes until the edges brown slightly; repeat process with remaining margarine and veal. Remove meat from pan and set it aside. To the pan drippings add three quarters of the lemon slices, the wine, and lemon juice; scrape drippings into this liquid, mix well and bring mixture to a boil. Return veal to pan and cook gently 2 to 3 minutes to blend flavors. Serve immediately on warmed platter. Garnish with remaining lemon slices and chopped parsley.

Nutritive values per serving: CHO 9 gm., PRO 28 gm., FAT 20 gm., Calories 323, Sodium 441 mg.

Food Exchanges per serving: 4 Medium-Fat Meat Exchanges plus 1 Fruit Exchange.

Low-sodium diets: Omit salt. Use unsalted margarine.

Veal Marengo

4 servings (yield: 12 ounces cooked
veal plus 2 cups vegetable gravy)

1 serving: 3 ounces
cooked veal plus ½ cup
vegetable gravy

1 pound fresh tomatoes
1 pound veal cutlets, about ¼ inch thick
2 tablespoons flour
½ teaspoon salt
¼ teaspoon pepper
2 tablespoons vegetable oil
¼ cup chopped onion
1 clove garlic, crushed
1 chicken bouillon cube
1 cup boiling water
¼ teaspoon grated lemon rind
½ teaspoon thyme
½ teaspoon oil (to oil pan)
¼ pound fresh mushrooms, sliced

Preheat oven to 350° F. (180° C.). Dip tomatoes in boiling water
for 10 seconds and remove skins; cut out cores; set tomatoes aside.
Cut cutlets in 4 or 8 equal-sized pieces. Measure into a small brown
paper bag 1 tablespoon flour, salt, and pepper; shake well. Add
pieces of veal. Hold top of bag together tightly with one hand, and
place other hand at bottom of bag; turn bag upside down and back
several times to coat all pieces evenly; set aside. Heat oil in a large
frying pan. Cook onion and garlic over medium heat, stirring until
onion is a light, golden color; remove carefully from oil and set aside.
Brown meat in hot oil turning with tongs frequently; remove meat
from pan. Add 1 tablespoon flour to pan and stir vigorously until
browned. Dissolve bouillon cube in boiling water, then add slowly to
flour in pan; continue stirring. Cook and stir over moderate heat until
thickened and smooth; add lemon rind, thyme, and onions; mix;
remove from heat. Slice tomatoes; arrange in the bottom of a lightly
oiled 1½-quart baking pan. Arrange meat on top, then cover with
brown sauce. Cover and bake 30 minutes. Add mushrooms and mix
into sauce. Bake uncovered 20 minutes more.

Nutritive values per serving: CHO 10 gm., PRO 25 gm., FAT 18 gm., Calories 302, Sodium 591 mg.

Food Exchanges per serving: 3 Medium-Fat Meat Exchanges plus 2 Vegetable Exchanges.

Low-sodium diets: Omit salt. Use low-sodium chicken bouillon cube.

LAMB

Roast Lamb

Roasting cuts of lamb include the leg, loin, and shoulder of lamb. All of these cuts may be boned at the market for easier carving. As with beef, do not roast a piece weighing less than 3 pounds.

Season lamb by inserting slivers of garlic into the meat with the tip of a sharp knife, sprinkle with coarse ground pepper, and rub with soy sauce. Or use your favorite herb seasonings, such as mint or dill.

Roast lamb at 325° F. (165° C.) 25 to 30 minutes per pound with the fat side up. A meat thermometer inserted into the thickest part of the meat should register 170° F. to 180° F. (70° C. to 80° C.) when lamb is done. Lamb usually takes 30 to 35 minutes per pound to cook. Rolled cuts take longer, about 45 minutes per pound.

Nutritive values per serving (3 ounces or 85 grams lean, boneless, cooked lamb, trimmed of fat: Leg of lamb—CHO 0, PRO 22 gm., FAT 16 gm., Calories 237, Sodium 53 mg.

Loin (saddle) of lamb—CHO 0, PRO 24 gm., FAT 6 gm., Calories 160, Sodium 59 mg.

Shoulder of lamb—CHO 0, PRO 23 gm., FAT 9 gm., Calories 174, Sodium 56 mg.

Food Exchanges per serving: Leg of lamb—3 Medium-Fat Meat Exchanges.

Loin or shoulder of lamb—3 Lean Meat Exchanges.

Low-sodium diets: Do not use salt or soy sauce in seasoning meat.

Shashlik

The meat in this recipe must marinate for 24 hours, so you must begin preparations the day before you are to serve this dish. This is sometimes called Shish Kebab and may be prepared with lean beef cubes if you prefer.

7 to 14 servings (yield: 14 skewers)   1 serving: 1 to 2 skewers

3¾ pounds lean leg of lamb, sirloin half
¼ cup olive oil
¼ cup wine vinegar
1 teaspoon basil
1 clove garlic, crushed
2 medium sweet green peppers, cored and cut into 1-inch cubes (about 1¼ cups)
2 medium onions, (about 8 ounces) each cut into 6 wedges
½ pound fresh mushrooms, cleaned
1 medium (about 4 to 5 ounces) sweet red pepper, cleaned and cut into 1-inch cubes

Have meat cutter remove bone, fat, and tendons, and cut the lamb into 1-inch cubes. The yield will be about 2 pounds (910 grams) lean lamb cubes. Place meat in medium-sized bowl. Combine the oil, vinegar, basil, and garlic. Pour over meat and mix well. Cover and place in the refrigerator for 24 hours, turning marinade through meat occasionally. Remove meat from refrigerator at least 1 hour before use; drain off all oil mixture. On 11-inch skewers thread alternating pieces of vegetables and meat (green pepper, meat, onion, red pepper, meat, mushroom, green pepper). Charcoal broil or oven broil kebabs for 5 minutes on each side or until meat is cooked but pink inside.

Nutritive values per serving:
    2 skewers—CHO 7 gm., PRO 39 gm., FAT 15 gm., Calories 325, Sodium 104 mg.
    1 skewer—CHO 4 gm., PRO 19 gm., FAT 8 gm., Calories 163, Sodium 52 mg.

Food Exchanges per serving:
    2 skewers—5 Lean Meat Exchanges plus 2 Vegetable Exchanges.
    1 skewer—2½ Lean Meat Exchanges plus 1 Vegetable Exchange.
Low-sodium diets: This recipe is suitable.

Lamb Curry

If you serve this delicious, traditional Lamb Curry with rice, don't forget to add the nutritive values and food exchanges.

6 servings (yield: 4½ cups)   1 serving: ¾ cup

2 tablespoons margarine
2 cups coarsely chopped onions
1 large clove garlic, minced
1½ pounds boneless lean lamb, cut into 1-inch cubes
3 tablespoons flour
1 tablespoon curry powder (Real curry lovers prefer 1½ tablespoons.)
¼ teaspoon ground ginger
1 teaspoon salt
1½ cups hot chicken broth
1 can (16 ounces) tomatoes
1 cup (100 grams) cubed, pared apple

Melt margarine in a large deep frying pan. Add onions, garlic, and lamb and cook over medium heat until meat is browned all over. Remove lamb and onions with a slotted spoon and set aside. Combine flour, curry powder, ginger, and salt and stir into remaining fat in frying pan; blend well. Add hot chicken broth slowly, stirring constantly, until smooth and beginning to bubble. Cut tomatoes in bite-sized pieces; add tomatoes with tomato liquid, lamb, onions, and apples to mixture in pan. Stir to blend; bring to a simmer. Cover and cook over low heat about 45 minutes or until meat is tender, stirring occasionally. Serve with plain boiled rice, Rice Pallau, or Rizzi Bizzi (*see* Index), and add on those food values.

Nutritive values per serving: CHO 15 gm., PRO 25 gm., FAT 10 gm., Calories 250, Sodium 742 mg.

Food Exchanges per serving: 1 Bread Exchange plus 3½ Lean Meat Exchanges.

Low-sodium diets: Omit salt. Use unsalted margarine, low-sodium chicken broth, and unsalted canned tomatoes.

PORK

Pork Roast

Lean pork from a young animal is a pale pink color. Meat from older animals is a darker pink. For roasting, choose a pork loin or shoulder or use a fresh ham.

Season the roast with (1) ginger and garlic, or (2) marjoram and salt, or (3) Dijon mustard and pepper, or (4) any combination of your favorite seasonings.

Place the roast on a rack in a shallow roasting pan with the fat side up. Roast at 350° F. (165° C.) until the meat is tender, about 35 minutes per pound. Insert a meat thermometer in the thickest part of the meat. Pork is done when the thermometer registers 170° F. (75° C.). Older cookbooks advise 185° F. (85° C.) but newer information suggests that that temperature is too high and makes the meat less palatable. The 170° F. (75°C.) temperature is perfectly safe.

If you want the roast to have a slightly glazed appearance, baste it during the last 15 or 20 minutes of cooking time with ⅓ cup unsweetened pineapple juice or apple juice. Serve with Granny Smith Applesauce, Sweet Pickled Cherries, or Raisins Indienne (*see* Index).

Nutritive values per serving
   (3 ounces cooked, boneless
   lean pork roast trimmed
   of fat):   CHO 0, PRO 25 gm., FAT 12 gm., Calories 216, Sodium 61 mg. (Calculations are based on ginger and garlic seasoning.)

Food Exchanges per serving
   of 3 ounces: 3 Medium-Fat Meat Exchanges.

Low-sodium diets: Do not use salt in seasoning pork roast. Also, choose an accompaniment low in sodium.

Basil Pork Chops

4 servings   1 serving: 1 chop plus 1 tablespoon sauce

4 lean center-cut pork chops (1¼ pounds)
1 cup V-8 Juice
1 teaspoon sweet basil
½ teaspoon salt
¼ teaspoon coarsely ground pepper

Trim and discard excess fat from chops. In a large frying pan, brown chops without added fat. When chops are browned, add other ingredients. Cover tightly and simmer 40 minutes or until tender. Turn meat occasionally, and add a few tablespoons of water if necessary to avoid burning.

Nutritive values per serving: CHO 2 gm., PRO 20 gm., FAT 23 gm., Calories 297, Sodium 401 gm.

Food Exchanges per serving: 3 High-Fat Meat Exchanges.

Low-sodium diets: Omit salt. Substitute unsalted tomato juice for the V-8.

Savory Loin Pork Chops

4 servings   1 serving: 1 chop

4 (2 pounds) loin pork chops, bone in
½ teaspoon salt
⅛ teaspoon marjoram
⅛ teaspoon thyme
⅛ teaspoon sage
¾ cup chicken broth
½ teaspoon grated orange rind
⅛ teaspoon ground ginger

Preheat oven to 300° F. (150° C.). Cut off fat around outside of all chops. Over medium heat partially cook some of the fat pieces in a heavy frying pan until there is about a tablespoon of liquid fat in pan. Discard all the rest of the fat. Combine salt, marjoram, thyme, and sage. Sprinkle on both sides of chops and press in with fingers. Brown chops on both sides in the frying pan, turning twice. Transfer to a shallow casserole. Combine chicken broth, orange rind, and ginger; pour over chops. Cover casserole. Bake 45 minutes, uncovering last 5 minutes of cooking.

Nutritive values per serving: CHO 0, PRO 29 gm., FAT 18 gm., Calories 285, Sodium 472 mg.

Food Exchanges per serving: 4 Medium-Fat Meat Exchanges. Purchase 1½ pounds of thinner chops to yield 3 Medium-Fat Meat Exchanges per serving.

Low-sodium diets: Omit salt. Use unsalted chicken broth.

Baked Ham

Precooked hams are widely available both in cans and in the meat display case of your local market. Place the ham on a rack in a shallow roasting pan. Score the surface of the ham and season with dry mustard powder and stud with whole cloves.

Heat precooked ham in a 325° F. (165° C.) oven for 10 to 15 minutes per pound of ham. According to the National Live Stock and Meat Board, "fully cooked," or precooked, hams should reach a temperature of 140° F. (60° C.) when they are heated for serving hot.

Trim ham of separable fat before serving. Serve with Mustard Sauce or Sweet and Sour Sauce (*see* Index). Add values of sauce to nutritive and exchange values below.

Nutritive values per serving
(3 ounces): CHO 0, PRO 24 gm., FAT 8 gm., Calories 179, Sodium 863 mg.

Food Exchanges per serving: 3 Lean Meat Exchanges.

Low-sodium diets: This recipe is not suitable.

Broiled Ham Steak

Choose a precooked center cut ham steak ½ inch thick. Cut ridges in the fat surrounding ham so that the edges will not curl. Brush each side with 1 teaspoon prepared mustard. Broil ham 3 inches from broiler heat for 3 minutes on each side. Trim fat from around outside edges and discard.

If you are using fresh ham, broil ham slice 3 inches from broiler heat for 7 to 8 minutes on each side.

Nutritive values per serving
(3 ounces): CHO 0, PRO 24 gm., FAT 9 gm., Calories 181, Sodium 895 mg.

Food Exchanges per serving: 3 Lean Meat Exchanges.

Low-sodium diets: This recipe is not suitable.

Baked Ham Loaf

4 servings   1 serving: a 1¾-inch thick slice

2 medium eggs, beaten
¼ cup catsup
1 tablespoon prepared mustard
½ cup skim milk
2¾ cups ground, cooked ham
2 slices fresh bread, finely crumbled
2 tablespoons finely cut onions
½ cup finely cut celery
3 tablespoons minced parsley

Preheat oven to 350° F. (180° C.). Prepare a 7½-by-3½-by-2-inch loaf pan or four 6-ounce custard cups with vegetable pan coating (solid or spray). Combine beaten eggs, catsup, mustard, and milk. Add all remaining ingredients; mix well. Turn into the loaf pan or custard cups. Bake 1 hour for loaf pan or 40 minutes for individual custard cups. Remove from oven and allow to stand for 5 minutes. Unmold on a serving platter. Cut loaf into four slices.

Nutritive values per serving: CHO 15 gm., PRO 22 gm., FAT 20 gm., Calories 329; Sodium 929 mg.

Food Exchanges per serving: 3 Medium-Fat Meat Exchanges plus 1 Bread Exchange plus ½ Fat Exchange.

Low-sodium diets: This recipe is not suitable.

Big Dawgs

Although Kay developed this one for young "kids," she found that "big kids" like it too—hence the name!

5 servings (yield: 10 frankfurters plus 1¼ cups sauce)

1 serving: 2 frankfurters plus ¼ cup sauce

¾ cup catsup
1 teaspoon chili powder
1 tablespoon Worcestershire sauce
1 cup water
1 teaspoon onion powder
10 fully cooked frankfurters (1 pound)

Combine all ingredients except frankfurters in a 10-inch frying pan; mix well and bring to a boil. Add frankfurters; simmer gently 15 to 20 minutes. If desired, serve on hot cooked rice or noodles.

Nutritive values per serving: CHO 12 gm., PRO 12 gm., FAT 25 gm., Calories 324, Sodium 1,545 mg. If served on ⅓ cup rice or noodles, add 68 calories and CHO 15 gm., PRO 2 gm.

Food Exchanges per serving: 2 High-Fat Meat Exchanges plus 2 Fat Exchanges plus 1 Fruit Exchange. If served on ⅓ cup hot rice or noodles add 1 Bread Exchange.

Low-sodium diets: This recipe is not suitable.

Knockwurst and Sauerkraut

5 servings   1 serving: 2 knockwurst plus ½ cup sauerkraut

2 teaspoons margarine
1 cup chopped onions
2 cans (16 ounces each) sauerkraut
1½ teaspoons caraway seed (optional)
10 knockwursts (2 packages, 12 ounces each)

Preheat oven to 350° F. (180° C.). Brown onions in margarine in a large frying pan. Add sauerkraut with its liquid and caraway seeds; heat together 3 to 4 minutes to blend flavors. Transfer mixture to a large flat casserole and top with knockwursts. Bake 20 to 25 minutes, turning knockwursts several times so that they brown as they cook.

Nutritive values per serving:
   2 knockwurst and ½ cup sauerkraut   —CHO 13 gm., PRO 21 gm., FAT 34 gm., Calories 438, Sodium 2,703 mg.

   1 knockwurst and ¼ cup sauerkraut   —CHO 7 gm., PRO 11 gm., FAT 17 gm., Calories 219, Sodium 1,351 mg.

Food Exchanges per serving:
   2 knockwurst and ½ cup sauerkraut   —1 Bread Exchange plus 3 High-Fat Meat Exchanges plus 2 Fat Exchanges.

   1 knockwurst and ¼ cup sauerkraut   —1 Vegetable Exchange plus 2 High-Fat Meat Exchanges.

Low-sodium diets: This recipe is not suitable.

29

Poultry

Roast Chicken or Capon

Select a plump meaty bird for roasting, either a young roasting chicken or capon. Clean and stuff the bird using Bread Stuffing (*see* Index). If bird is very fat, remove and discard separable fat in body cavity. Tie legs securely.

Place bird breast side up on a rack in an open roasting pan. Rub skin with margarine. Cover bird loosely with foil. Roast at 325°F. (165° C.) until tender (2½ to 3 hours for a 4-pound bird). Thirty minutes before the roasting time is up, remove foil and baste with drippings so that the skin will brown. When bird is done the drumstick will twist easily. Let bird stand 15 minutes after removal from oven for easier carving.

Nutritive values per serving 3½ ounces, or 100 grams, boneless roasted chicken with attached skin plus ½ cup Bread Stuffing: CHO 17 gm., PRO 30 gm., FAT 10 gm., Calories 281, Sodium 478 mg.

Food Exchanges per serving: 4 Lean Meat Exchanges plus 1 Bread Exchange.

Low-sodium diets: Rub bird with unsalted margarine. Bread Stuffing is not suitable; substitute a stuffing low in sodium.

Stewed Chicken

Sometimes we want cooked chicken to use in salads, in sandwich fillings, for cold, sliced chicken, and in casserole dishes. It's a good idea to buy stewing chickens when they are available because they are the most flavorful kind for cooking in water. They are usually larger than roasters or fryers. Whatever kind you get, have it cut up into pieces, including the neck but excluding the giblets.

When stewing chickens are not available, select the largest whole or cut-up chicken you can find. Place chicken in a large, deep kettle. For every 1 pound of chicken pieces, add ½ to 1 cup water and ½ teaspoon salt. For added flavor also add to water ½ cup sliced carrot, ½ cup sliced onion, 1 or 2 stalks of celery cut up with leaves, and 1 dried red pepper pod, 1 to 2 inches long (no larger). Bring to a rapid boil and remove any froth from surface. Cover the pot, reduce heat, and let simmer gently until the thickest parts of the chicken are fork-tender, which will be 2½ to 4 hours. The cooking time depends upon the age and the size of the chicken. Remove kettle from heat. With tongs, lift chicken pieces out carefully and place in a large shallow pan to cool quickly. Strain liquid, discard vegetables, and pour liquid into jars; cool, cover, and chill. When cold, the fat may be removed easily from the surface.

Cool the chicken as quickly as possible. Separate the good white and dark meat from the skin, bones, and gristle; discard these inedible parts. Wrap cooked chicken meat in plastic wrap or bags and store in refrigerator. Do not slice or dice the chicken until ready to use in a recipe or ready to serve.

The strained cooking liquid, when chilled, may form a gel, which will make a delicious jellied chicken consommé. Or it may be used as a base (diluted with some water) to make chicken soup, a sauce or gravy, or used in recipes calling for chicken broth.

Nutritive values per serving:
(1 ounce cooked chicken meat):   CHO 0, PRO 9 gm., FAT 2 gm., Calories 55, Sodium 16 mg. Salt added in cooking water must be added to this value.

Food Exchange per 1 ounce cooked·   1 Lean Meat Exchange.

Low-sodium diets: Omit salt in cooking water.

Baked Chicken Barbecue

4 servings   1 serving: ½ breast and wing plus ¼ cup sauce
                              or 1 leg and 1 thigh plus ¼ cup sauce

1 whole chicken (2½ pounds), cut up
1 cup Barbecue Sauce (*see* Index)

Prepare the Barbecue Sauce. Preheat oven to 400° F. (205° C.).
Line bottom and sides of a shallow baking pan with foil or prepare
pan with vegetable pan coating (spray or solid). Baste each chicken
piece with sauce. Arrange chicken pieces in pan with skin sides up;
pour remaining sauce evenly on top. Cover pan with foil; bake 45
minutes; uncover pan, and bake for another 20 minutes.

Nutritive values per serving: CHO 10 gm., PRO 32 gm., FAT 10
                                 gm., Calories 262, Sodium 361 mg.

Food Exchanges per serving: 4 Lean Meat Exchanges plus 1 Fruit
                               Exchange.

Low-sodium diets: Modify Barbecue Sauce recipe as directed.

Chicken Cacciatore

4 servings

1 serving: ½ breast and wing plus ½ cup tomato mixture *or* 1 leg and 1 thigh plus ½ cup tomato mixture

1 chicken (2½ pounds), cut in pieces
1 tablespoon vegetable oil
½ cup chopped onions
½ cup finely cut strips of sweet green pepper
1 can (16 ounces) tomatoes, cut up, with liquid
⅓ cup tomato paste
¾ teaspoon salt
⅛ teaspoon garlic powder
½ teaspoon crushed oregano
⅛ teaspoon allspice
¼ cup lemon juice
½ cup water

Preheat oven to 400° F. (205° C.). Prepare a large casserole with vegetable pan coating (spray or solid). Wipe chicken pieces with damp cloth. Heat vegetable oil in a large frying pan. Brown chicken pieces on both sides; transfer to casserole. Cook onions and pepper strips in frying pan for 3 to 4 minutes, stirring frequently. Combine tomatoes with all remaining ingredients and mix well; add to onions and green peppers. Bring to a boil. Pour evenly on top of chicken. Bake 30 minutes. Turn chicken over and baste with sauce; bake 20 to 30 minutes more until chicken is tender.

Nutritive values per serving: CHO 15 gm., PRO 33 gm., FAT 13 gm., Calories 313, Sodium 690 mg.

Food Exchanges per serving: 4½ Lean Meat Exchanges plus 1 Bread Exchange.

Low-sodium diets: Omit salt. Use unsalted canned tomatoes and unsalted tomato paste.

Lemon Chicken

Lemon Chicken is shown on the cover of this book. Pretty, isn't it? And it's delicious cold for picnics or on a buffet.

4 servings   1 serving: 1 leg and thigh *or* ½ breast and wing

1 frying chicken (2½ pounds), cut in pieces
1 teaspoon salt
¼ teaspoon pepper
¼ teaspoon garlic powder
1 teaspoon basil
⅓ cup lemon juice
¼ cup water
1½ teaspoons grated lemon peel
3 to 4 thin slices of lemon for garnish

Preheat oven to 400° F. (205° C.). Cut chicken breast in half. Sprinkle chicken pieces with salt, pepper, and garlic. Place pieces in a shallow baking pan with skin side down. Combine remaining ingredients except lemon slices and pour over chicken. Bake, uncovered, for 20 minutes. Turn chicken and baste with pan drippings. Bake for 30 to 40 minutes more until chicken is tender. Serve on a platter garnished with lemon slices.

Nutritive values per serving: CHO 4 gm., PRO 31 gm., FAT 10 gm., Calories 233, Sodium 616 mg.

Food Exchanges per serving: 4½ Lean Meat Exchanges plus ½ Fruit Exchange.

Low-sodium diets: Omit salt.

Chicken a la King

4 servings (yield: 2⅔ cups)   1 serving: ⅔ cup

2 tablespoons margarine
¼ cup flour
1¼ cups chicken broth
1 cup skim milk
⅛ teaspoon pepper
¼ teaspoon paprika
½ teaspoon salt
1 teaspoon minced onion
⅛ teaspoon ginger
1¾ cup diced, cooked chicken, without skin
1 can (3½ to 4 ounces) button mushrooms, drained
1½ tablespoons finely diced pimiento

Melt margarine in a large saucepan. Stir in flour, mixing until smooth. Add chicken broth and milk gradually, stirring constantly. Cook and stir over medium heat until thick and smooth. Add pepper, paprika, salt, onion, and ginger; stir to mix well. Add chicken and mushrooms and stir over low heat for 5 minutes. Add pimiento, stir over heat about 2 to 3 minutes, then serve. If served over toast, baking powder biscuits, or noodles, remember to add the additional nutritive values and Food Exchanges.

Nutritive values per serving: CHO 10 gm., PRO 24 gm., FAT 8 gm., Calories 215, Sodium 733 mg.

Food Exchanges per serving: 3½ Lean Meat Exchanges plus ½ Bread Exchange.

Low-sodium diets: Omit salt. Use unsalted margarine, unsalted chicken broth, and unsalted canned mushrooms.

Chicken Chow Mein

6 servings (yield: 6 cups)   1 serving: 1 cup chicken-vegetable mixture
plus about ⅓ cup chow mein noodles

1 tablespoon vegetable oil
3 cups slant-sliced celery
½ cup slant-sliced green onions, with tops
2½ cups hot chicken broth
3 tablespoons cornstarch
½ teaspoon salt
⅛ teaspoon garlic powder or 1 clove garlic, minced
½ teaspoon ground ginger
½ cup cold water
1 tablespoon soy sauce
3¼ cups firmly packed, cooked chicken, cut into bite-sized pieces
1¼ cups sweet green pepper, cut into 1-inch cubes
1 can (6 ounces) mushroom stems and pieces, drained
1 can (8 ounces) water chestnuts, drained and sliced
1 can (3½ ounces) chow mein noodles
2 tablespoons finely cut candied ginger

Heat vegetable oil in a deep, heavy cooking pot; add celery and onions; stir-fry over moderate heat until onions are transparent but not brown. Add chicken broth, cover and cook over low heat 4 to 5 minutes. Meanwhile, combine cornstarch, salt, garlic, ginger, cold water, and soy sauce and mix until smooth. Add slowly to hot mixture, stirring constantly. Cook and stir over medium heat until liquid thickens and is clear. Add chicken, green pepper, mushrooms, and water chestnuts; mix well. Cover and let cook over low heat about 5 minutes until heated throughout. To serve, turn into a 2-quart serving dish. Mix noodles and candied ginger and scatter on top of chicken mixture.

Nutritive values per serving: CHO 27 gm., PRO 32 gm., FAT 11 gm., Calories 329, Sodium 971 mg.

Food Exchanges per serving
(includes noodles):   1 Bread Exchange plus 2 Vegetable Exchanges plus 3½ Low-Fat Meat Exchanges.

Low-sodium diets: Omit salt. Substitute low-sodium Worcestershire sauce for soy sauce, and fresh mushrooms for canned mushrooms, and use unsalted chicken broth.

Ginger Chicken and Vegetables

4 servings (yield: 4 cups)   1 serving: 1 cup

3 tablespoons soy sauce
1 tablespoon cornstarch
⅓ cup water
1 tablespoon dry sherry
1 teaspoon grated fresh ginger root
¾ pound boned chicken breasts
1 tablespoon vegetable oil
1 medium onion, sliced in wedges (¼ pound)
¾ cup slant-sliced celery
¼ pound fresh mushrooms, sliced
¼ pound fresh spinach, cleaned and torn

Prepare a marinade of soy sauce, cornstarch, water, dry sherry, and ginger. Cut chicken in thin strips and soak in marinade 20 minutes. Meanwhile, clean and cut the vegetables. Heat oil in a very large frying pan. Drain the chicken and reserve the marinade; sauté chicken in oil 2 minutes. Add onions and celery and stir-fry for 3 more minutes. Stir in the mushrooms; mix well. Add the spinach, stir-fry 2 minutes; add reserved marinade and heat through. Serve immediately.

Nutritive values per serving: CHO 11 gm., PRO 26 gm., FAT 8 gm., Calories 234, Sodium 1,103 mg.

Food Exchanges per serving: 3 Lean Meat Exchanges plus 2 Vegetable Exchanges.

Low-sodium diets: Substitute low-sodium Worcestershire sauce for the soy sauce. Add 1 additional tablespoon dry sherry.

Chicken Paprika

4 servings (yield: 1⅓ cups of the vegetables and gravy, plus the chicken pieces)

1 serving: ½ breast and wing plus ⅓ cup vegetable gravy *or* 1 leg and thigh plus ⅓ cup vegetable gravy

1 chicken (2½ pounds), cut in pieces
2 tablespoons olive oil
1 clove garlic, crushed
1 cup chopped onion
1½ tablespoons paprika (more or less, as desired)
½ teaspoon ground cumin
2 cups chicken broth
½ teaspoon salt
1 cup cross-sliced carrots
2 tablespoons tomato paste

Wipe chicken pieces with a damp paper towel and set aside. Heat oil in a deep, 10- or 12-inch frying pan. Add garlic and onion and cook gently over low heat, stirring occasionally, until they are a very light golden color. Add paprika and cumin and continue cooking about 1 minute. Place chicken pieces in pan with skin side down. Add chicken broth, salt, and carrots; cover pan tightly and simmer over low heat for 25 minutes. Stir in the tomato paste. Turn chicken pieces, cover again, and simmer over low heat for 25 to 30 minutes or until chicken is tender.

Nutritive values per serving: CHO 10 gm., PRO 34 gm., FAT 17 gm., Calories 336, Sodium 786 mg.

Food Exchanges per serving: 4 Lean Meat Exchanges plus 2 Vegetable Exchanges plus 1 Fat Exchange.

Low-sodium diets: Omit salt. Use unsalted chicken broth and unsalted tomato paste.

Java Chicken

4 servings   1 serving: ½ breast and
                                              wing *or* 1 leg and thigh

⅓ cup flour
2 teaspoons coarsely ground pepper
1 teaspoon salt
1 chicken (2½ pounds), cut up
2 tablespoons margarine
1 tablespoon vegetable oil
1 cup skim milk

In a small brown bag combine flour, pepper, and salt. Coat chicken pieces, one at a time, by shaking in the bag. Fold the top of the bag to contain the flour mixture while shaking. Reserve remaining flour mixture. Heat margarine and oil in a large frying pan; brown the chicken. Cover pan, reduce heat, and cook 30 to 40 minutes until done. Remove chicken from pan; stir remaining flour mixture (about 2 tablespoons) into pan drippings. Slowly add milk and stir until gravy is thickened. Pour gravy over chicken before serving. If you serve mashed potatoes, cooked noodles, or Rizzi Bizzi (*see* Index) with this recipe, be sure to add the nutritive values and Food Exchanges for whichever you choose.

Nutritive values per serving: CHO 14 gm., PRO 34 gm., FAT 20 gm., Calories 371, Sodium 718 mg.

Food Exchanges per serving: 4½ Medium-Fat Meat Exchanges plus 1 Bread Exchange.

Low-sodium diets: Omit salt. Use unsalted margarine.

Mideast Chicken

This makes an attractive dinner when served with a bright green vegetable or salad.

4 servings

1 serving: ½ chicken breast plus ⅓ cup cooked bulgur

2 tablespoons vegetable oil
¼ cup finely chopped onion
½ cup thinly sliced carrots
⅛ teaspoon dried dill weed
¼ teaspoon ground ginger
½ teaspoon curry powder
1/16 teaspoon ground cardamom
½ teaspoon cinnamon
1 teaspoon salt
1½ pounds chicken breasts (2 whole or 4 halves)
½ cup finely cut sweet green pepper
2 chicken bouillon cubes
2 cups boiling water
½ teaspoon paprika
⅓ cup bulgur

Heat oil in a large, deep, 12-inch frying pan. Add onions, carrots, dill, ginger, curry, cardamom, cinnamon, and salt; cook over moderate heat stirring with a wooden spoon until onions are tender. Meanwhile, split whole chicken breasts; add to cooking vegetable mixture and brown halves on both sides, turning with tongs. When lightly browned, add green pepper, chicken bouillon cubes, boiling water, and paprika; mix carefully. Simmer covered for 20 minutes. Add bulgur carefully; bring to a boil again, cover, and simmer gently for 20 to 25 minutes or until bulgur is tender. Check pan occasionally to prevent mixture from boiling dry; if necessary add a little boiling water.

Nutritive values per serving: CHO 15 gm., PRO 28 gm., FAT 12 gm., Calories 281, Sodium 1088 mg.

Food Exchanges per serving: 1 Bread Exchange plus 4 Lean Meat Exchanges.

Low-sodium diets: Omit salt. Use low-sodium chicken bouillon cubes.

Dijon Chicken

4 servings   1 serving: ½ breast plus 2
                                                    tablespoons sauce

2 whole chicken breasts, without skin or bones
2 tablespoons margarine
2 cloves garlic, crushed
½ cup dry white wine
¼ cup water
2 tablespoons Dijon mustard
½ teaspoon dried dill weed
½ teaspoon salt
¼ teaspoon coarsely ground black pepper
¼ cup chopped fresh parsley

Preheat oven to 325°F. (165°C.). Cut each boned breast into two
pieces; put pieces on a wooden cutting board and pound them with a
meat mallet or the side of a rolling pin until ½ inch thick. Heat
margarine in a large frying pan; add garlic and cook 2 minutes over
medium heat. Brown chicken pieces 3 minutes on each side. Transfer
chicken to a 1½-quart shallow casserole dish. Put the wine, water,
mustard, dill weed, salt, and pepper into the frying pan; stir to mix
with the chicken drippings in the pan. Bring to a boil and cook 1
minute. Pour over chicken in casserole. Cover and bake 30 minutes.
Add parsley; baste the chicken with the sauce and cook 5 more
minutes.

Nutritive values per serving: CHO 4 gm., PRO 31 gm., FAT 12
                                 gm., Calories 256, Sodium 502 mg.

Food Exchanges per serving: 4 Lean Meat Exchanges plus 1
                                 Vegetable Exchange.

Low-sodium diets: Omit salt. Use unsalted margarine.

Chicken Cantonese

6 servings (yield: 4½ cups)   1 serving: ¾ cup

1¼ pounds chicken breast, without bones or skin
1 tablespoon vegetable oil
½ cup slant-sliced celery
¼ cup sliced green onions
1 clove garlic, minced
1¼ cups chicken bouillon
1 teaspoon salt
½ teaspoon ginger
$\frac{1}{16}$ teaspoon pepper
1 cup sweet green pepper, cut into 2-inch squares
1 package (6 ounces) frozen Chinese pea pods
1 tablespoon cornstarch
¼ cup cold water

Cut boned and skinned chicken breasts into 2-by-½-inch strips. Heat oil in a large, deep skillet. Stir-fry celery, onions, garlic, and chicken strips over medium heat 3 to 4 minutes, turning the ingredients frequently with a large wooden spoon or fork. Add chicken bouillon, salt, ginger, and pepper; cover and bring to a boil. Add green pepper and Chinese pea pods; cover and cook over medium heat 6 to 8 minutes or until green pepper and pea pods are crisp-tender. Meanwhile, combine cornstarch and cold water; stir cornstarch mixture into skillet. Cook over medium heat until thick and clear, stirring constantly.

Nutritive values per serving: CHO 7 gm., PRO 31 gm., FAT 8 gm., Calories 235, Sodium 675 mg.

Food Exchanges per serving: 4 Lean Meat Exchanges plus 1 Vegetable Exchange.

Low-sodium diets: Omit salt. Use low-sodium chicken bouillon.

Spicy Szechwan Chicken

This is Peter's favorite recipe in the whole book! Be sure to have all ingredients sliced or diced and measured before you start the stir-fry cooking. Warning, this recipe is delicious but HOT!

6 servings (yield: 4 cups)   1 serving: ⅔ cup

1 pound boned and skinned chicken breasts
4 teaspoons cornstarch
1 egg white, unbeaten
2 tablespoons vegetable oil
¾ cup drained, canned bamboo shoots, thinly sliced
¼ cup drained, diced green chiles
½ cup shelled, roasted, skinned peanuts
1 clove garlic, finely minced
1 teaspoon sugar (Don't worry, it's OK.)
2 tablespoons soy sauce
3 tablespoons dry sherry
1 teaspoon grated, peeled ginger root
1 tablespoon finely chopped green onion

Cut chicken into 2-by-½-inch strips. Place in a large pie plate. Sprinkle 2 teaspoons cornstarch over chicken and mix well to coat chicken. Add egg white and mix again. Heat oil in a large 12-inch frying pan. Add chicken and bamboo shoots and stir-fry about 3 minutes (use a wooden spoon or wooden fork). Add chiles and peanuts; stir-fry 2 minutes. Combine all remaining ingredients except the green onions with 2 teaspoons cornstarch and add to the pan. Stir-fry and heat until sauce is thick and smooth and mixture is well blended. Add green onions. Stir-fry ½ minute to warm onions. Serve immediately.

Nutritive values per serving: CHO 8 gm., PRO 25 gm., FAT 15 gm., Calories 272, Sodium 554 mg. (estimated).

Food Exchanges per serving: 3½ Medium-Fat Meat Exchanges plus 1 Vegetable Exchange. When served on or with cooked rice, be sure to add 1 Bread Exchange per ⅓ cup rice, CHO 15 gm., PRO 2 gm., and Calories 68.

Low-sodium diets: This recipe is not suitable.

Chicken Breasts with Orange Sauce

4 servings (yield: 4 pieces chicken
plus 1 cup sauce)

1 serving: ½ breast plus
¼ cup sauce

2 whole chicken breasts, cut in half, or 1 chicken (2½ pounds),
cut in pieces
2 tablespoons margarine
1 teaspoon salt
⅛ teaspoon paprika
⅛ teaspoon ginger
1 tablespoon flour
1 cup chicken broth
¼ cup orange juice
2 thin slices orange with rind, cut crosswise
2 tablespoons finely cut candied ginger
1½ teaspoons grated, fresh orange rind

Preheat oven to 325° F. (165° C.). Melt margarine in a large skillet.
Brown chicken breasts in skillet over medium heat turning 2 or 3
times. Transfer chicken to a shallow casserole, skin side up; set aside.
Add seasonings and flour to hot fat in the skillet and stir to blend
until smooth and lightly browned. Gradually add chicken broth and
orange juice, stirring constantly. Cook and stir over low heat until
smooth and thickened. Pour on top of chicken; bake 30 minutes. Cut
each orange slice in quarters, and place two quarter slices on top of
each piece of chicken. Scatter ginger and grated orange rind on top.
Bake another 10 to 15 minutes.

Nutritive values per serving:	CHO 12 gm., PRO 27 gm., FAT 11 gm., Calories 259, Sodium 849 mg.
Food Exchanges per serving:	4 Lean Meat Exchanges plus 1 Fruit Exchange.
Low-sodium diets:	Omit salt. Use unsalted margarine and unsalted chicken broth.

Jellied Chicken Mold

5 servings (yield: 3½ cups)

1 serving: ⅔ cup
plus 2 teaspoons
regular mayonnaise

1½ tablespoons granulated gelatin
½ cup cold water
2¼ cups hot chicken broth
1 tablespoon lemon juice
1½ cups finely cut cooked chicken
¼ cup finely chopped celery
2 tablespoons finely chopped black olives
2 tablespoons finely chopped green onions
2 tablespoons diced pimientos
10 teaspoons regular mayonnaise

Soak gelatin in cold water. Add very hot chicken broth and lemon juice; stir to dissolve. Cool and then chill in the refrigerator until mixture is of the consistency of unbeaten egg whites. Carefully fold in all remaining ingredients except the mayonnaise. Turn into a 4-cup ring mold, a 7½-by-3¾-by-2-inch loaf pan, or five 6-ounce individual molds. Cover with plastic wrap. Chill about 3 hours before unmolding. If molded in a loaf pan, unmold, cut in 5 slices about 1½ inches thick, and place 2 teaspoons regular mayonnaise on top of each serving. If molded in a 4-cup ring mold, unmold onto crisp lettuce and place a small bowl with mayonnaise in the center of the ring.

Nutritive values per serving:*   CHO 2 gm., PRO 20 gm., FAT 10 gm., Calories 165, Sodium 409 mg.

Food Exchanges per serving:*   3 Lean Meat Exchanges.

Low-sodium diets: Use low-sodium broth and low-sodium mayonnaise.

* The nutritive values of the mayonnaise are calculated into the recipe. The calories and fat indicated above includes fat and calories from the mayonnaise. The protein value of chicken is high but the fat value of chicken is even lower than that in a Lean Meat Exchange. So the regular mayonnaise is a free bonus. Do not count additional Fat Exchanges for it.

Lean Chicken Gravy

Use recipe for Lean Beef Gravy (*see* Index), but in place of the beef bouillon cubes use chicken bouillon cubes. Yield, servings, nutritive values, Food Exchanges, and low-sodium recipe directions are the same.

Roast Turkey

Today's meat markets generally have a choice of frozen, stuffed, and unstuffed turkeys. The packages give clear, easy-to-follow directions for thawing, roasting temperatures, and cooking times depending upon the size of the bird. You may use prestuffed turkeys but we remind you that our Bread Stuffing (*see* Index) is much lower in calorie and fat values than commercial stuffings. Yet it is delicious for the entire family. The full recipe is ample for a 5 to 6 pound bird, so double the recipe for a 10 to 12 pound bird or triple it for a very large turkey. The amount of stuffing needed can be based on ½ cup prepared stuffing for each pound of turkey.

There is no "must" rule about stuffing any poultry. If you want to cook turkey or chicken unstuffed, go ahead! With a damp cloth, simply wipe out the body cavity and season it lightly as desired. Fold the piece of neck skin up and over the top end of the back and fasten it with a skewer. Either tie the legs together over the body opening or tuck them into that band of skin under the tail. When preparing turkey for roasting, remove and discard any separable fat from around and under skin near the body cavity, just as you do when preparing a chicken.

When your bird is ready for roasting, place it on a rack in a shallow roasting pan. Spread a few tablespoons of softened margarine around the sides and top of bird. Cover the roasting pan with a tent of heavy-duty foil and place in oven preheated to 325° F. (165° C.). About 45 minutes before cooking time is completed, remove the tent of foil and baste bird.

The following roasting times are based on a preheated oven and on the bird being at room temperature:

Whole Turkey (Stuffed)	*Pounds*	*Approximate Cooking Times*
For unstuffed birds, reduce cooking time by about ½ hour.	6–8	3–3½ hours
	8–12	3½–4½ hours
	12–16	4½–5½ hours
	16–20	5½–6½ hours
	20–24	6½–7 hours

Turkey (Halves or quarters)	*Pounds*	*Approximate Cooking Times*
	3–8	2–3 hours
	8–12	3–4 hours

If the poultry is to be cooked from the frozen state, then extra time must be allowed to make sure the meat is completely cooked to be safe to eat as well as tasty. Unless the package directions state otherwise, commercially frozen stuffed poultry should not be thawed before cooking.

It is wise to plan the cooking time so that the bird will be done about 15 to 30 minutes before serving. Roast turkey can be carved much more easily after it has been at room temperature for this period.

Never store cooked turkey with stuffing inside it. If there is leftover turkey and stuffing, remove the stuffing and store it separately. Wipe out the inside of the cooked turkey before refrigerating. This will guard against food poisoning.

Nutritive values per serving
(3 ounces roast turkey, white and dark meat, excluding stuffing):
CHO 0, PRO 27 gm., FAT 5 gm., Calories 162, Sodium 111 mg.

Food Exchanges per serving:
3½ Lean Meat Exchanges. Because fat value is even lower than a Lean Meat Exchange, you may have some turkey skin or 2 tablespoons regularly prepared turkey gravy without using any of your Fat Exchanges at that meal. If you want more gravy, use recipe for Lean Chicken Gravy (*see* Index) and use ¼ cup "free."

Low-sodium diets:
Do not season turkey with any salt. Use unsalted margarine. Bread Stuffing is not suitable; substitute a stuffing low in sodium.

Rock Cornish Hens with Grapes

4 servings (yield: 2 hens plus
1 cup sauce)

1 serving: ½ hen plus
¼ cup sauce

1½ tablespoons margarine
1 teaspoon salt
¼ teaspoon pepper
2 Rock Cornish hens, 1¼ pounds each, thawed
½ cup chicken broth
½ cup dry white wine
¼ cup grape juice, unsweetened
½ cup seedless grapes, cut in half

Preheat oven to 350°F. (180°C.). Melt margarine in a saucepan; add salt and pepper. Split hens and place in a shallow baking pan, skin side up. Baste with margarine mixture. Roast hens in uncovered pan for 1¼ to 1½ hours, or until tender and browned; baste them several times with drippings. When hens are done, remove them from pan. Pour pan drippings into a small saucepan and add chicken broth, wine, and grape juice. Simmer 15 minutes or until volume is reduced to ¾ cup. Add grapes and cook 2 minutes over moderate heat.

Nutritive values per serving: CHO 8 gm., PRO 25 gm., FAT 8 gm., Calories 206, Sodium 744 mg.

Food Exchanges per serving: 3 Lean Meat Exchanges plus 1 Fruit Exchange.

Low-sodium diets: Omit salt. Use unsalted margarine and unsalted chicken broth.

Roast Duckling

4 servings

1 serving: 3½ ounces (100 grams) boneless duck meat plus ¼ cup sauce

1 duckling, 4½ to 5 pounds, fresh, or frozen and thawed
1 lemon, quartered lengthwise
1 medium apple, quartered
1 medium onion, quartered
2 cups water
1 cup Sweet and Sour Sauce (*see* Index)
1 tablespoon grated orange rind
1 thin slice orange, cut in quarters for garnish

Preheat oven to 400°F. (205°C.). Wash duckling and remove and discard any separable fat around and under skin. Remove any pinfeathers. Rub duckling all over, inside and out, with quartered lemon, squeezing juice at the same time. Place apple and onion pieces inside body cavity. (These are to be discarded before eating and are only used for flavoring.) With a two-tined kitchen fork, pierce skin of duckling all over in 10 to 15 places to allow fat to drain out. Place duck on rack in a shallow roasting pan. Pour water into bottom of pan at one corner of pan. Roast duckling uncovered for 1½ hours. Again, prick skin with fork in many places. Reduce oven heat to 350°F. (180°C.) and roast another 45 minutes. Meanwhile prepare 1 cup of Sweet and Sour Sauce, using ½ of that recipe. Add grated orange rind to the sauce. Serve the sauce with the duckling. Garnish the duckling with orange slices. Discard apples and onion after duck is carved.

Nutritive values per serving: CHO 7 gm., PRO 24 gm., FAT 24 gm., Calories 335, Sodium 412 mg. If you eat the skin, be sure to add 5 gm. FAT and 45 calories for each additional Fat Exchange.

Food Exchanges per serving: 3 High-Fat Meat Exchanges plus ½ Bread Exchange. If you eat the skin, be sure to add 1 or 2 Fat Exchanges.

Low-sodium diets: Omit Sweet and Sour Sauce and substitute Cooked Cranberry Sauce (*see* Index).

30
Fish

Cooking Fish

There are a few things to remember about the cooking of fish:

- Because fish has very little connective tissue it does not take long to cook.
- Overcooking fish always toughens it, so follow directions closely and watch the cooking time.
- The best tests for "cooked right" fish are: (1) the flesh flakes easily when pierced with a fork; (2) the flesh loses its translucent look and becomes opaque.
- Serve fish as soon after cooking as possible. It always tastes best when piping hot!

Baking is an especially suitable method for cooking fish. It can be used for cleaned whole fish, fish fillets, or fish steaks. The recipe for World's Fastest Fish in this chapter is a fine example of baking fillets. There are also several other recipes for baking fish.

The Foil-Baked Fish recipe is really a combination of *oven-*

cooking and *steaming.* The fish makes its own sauce, comes out tender and full of flavor, and the pan is so clean!

Poaching fish is a method of cooking fish gently in liquid, usually in either a seasoned water or milk. It is very simple, and again it results in a tasty fish. Try our recipe for Poached Fish.

Fish may also be prepared by *steaming* over boiling water. You may use a strainer with little "legs" that will sit above boiling water, or buy a regulation steamer for fish. Some cooks like to use their vegetable steamer for shrimp, scallops, fish steaks, or thick fillets cut into 2-inch cubes. Fish may even be tied in a cheesecloth bag for ease of handling. When steaming fish, don't let the water touch the fish, but do remember to cover the pot tightly. Generally, fish should be steamed for 10 minutes per inch thickness of **fish**—twice as long if fish is frozen.

Broiling is also an acceptable method of cooking some fish, such as small whole fish or fish sticks.

We have not included any recipes for *deep-fat frying* of fish. Diabetics are usually advised not to deep fry foods unless caloric needs are particularly high. The methods we have used in this book result in such good tasting fish dishes we hope you will try them all.

From a nutrition standpoint fish is a winner. Most varieties are very low in fat and high in protein and all are counted as Lean Meat Exchanges. Because most types of fish have so little fat you can safely eat some additional fat at the same meal without using up Fat Exchanges. Our recipes indicate this. In addition, the fat of fish is unsaturated and eating fish is highly encouraged by the American Heart Association and others concerned about your serum cholesterol.

Poached Fish

Use this method to poach any fish fillets or salmon steaks.

6 servings   1 serving: 3½ ounces

1½ pounds fresh or frozen perch fillets, thawed
2 cups water
3 tablespoons white vinegar
¼ cup finely cut onions
3 whole peppercorns
2 sprigs fresh parsley or dill
1 bay leaf, crushed
¼ teaspoon salt

Cut fish into six serving portions and place them in a large frying pan. Combine all other ingredients and add to pan. Bring to a boil; cover pan and reduce heat to low. Simmer 6 to 8 minutes or until fish flakes easily with a fork. Lift fish out of liquid carefully with a pancake turner. Serve with lemon wedges or with Sunshine Sauce, Cucumber Sauce, or Dill Sauce (*see* Index).

Nutritive values per serving: CHO 1 gm., PRO 22 gm., FAT 5 gm., Calories 140, Sodium 90 mg.

Food Exchanges per serving: 3 Lean Meat Exchanges. Because poached fish has even less fat than allowed in the Lean Meat Exchanges, feel free to use 1 teaspoon of a sauce or lemon butter over each serving without counting the Fat Exchange for the butter.

Low-sodium diets: Omit salt.

Foil-Baked Fish Fillets

3 servings   1 serving: 1 foil package of fish
                                                      (about 4 ounces cooked)

1 pound fresh or frozen fish fillets, thawed
1½ teaspoons vegetable oil (to oil foil)
1½ teaspoons lemon juice
1 tablespoon finely chopped onion
1 tablespoon finely chopped celery and leaves
⅛ teaspoon salt
Dash of pepper
1 tablespoon vegetable oil

Preheat oven to 400° F. (205° C.). Cut fresh or thawed fillets into 3 individual serving pieces. Tear or cut 3 separate pieces of heavy-duty foil about 12 or 14 inches square. Brush with 1½ teaspoons vegetable oil to coat centers of each piece of foil. Place fish on top of oiled areas, then sprinkle fish with lemon juice. On top of fish spread a layer of each: onion, celery, salt, and pepper. Sprinkle 1 tablespoon vegetable oil over all. Lift foil up from opposite sides of fish to come together across top; fold over twice then pinch together to seal tightly. Seal ends in same way. Place foil packages in a shallow pan. Bake 25 minutes. To serve, lift each package onto a dinner plate, unwrap, and transfer cooked fish and sauce with a wide pancake turner.

Nutritive values per serving: CHO 1 gm., PRO 29 gm., FAT 17
                                                gm., Calories 277, Sodium 171 mg.

Food Exchanges per serving: 4 Lean Meat Exchanges.

Low-sodium diets: Omit salt. Choose a freshwater fish.

World's Fastest Fish!

4 servings   1 serving: 3½ ounces

1 pound low-fat fish fillets (walleye   pike, sole, flounder, whitefish)
½ teaspoon vegetable oil (to prepare pan)
1 cup milk
1 teaspoon salt
24 saltine crackers, finely crushed
1 tablespoon vegetable oil
Lemon wedges

Preheat oven to 500° F. (260° C.). Lightly oil baking pan and set aside. Cut fish fillets into four serving pieces. Mix milk and salt together. Turn cracker crumbs into a large pie plate. Dip each piece of fish into milk, then crumbs, then milk, then crumbs again to coat thoroughly and place fish pieces in the oiled baking pan. Liberally sprinkle 1 tablespoon of oil all over tops of fish pieces. Bake 10 to 12 minutes or until fish flakes lightly with a fork. Serve with wedges of lemon.

Nutritive values per serving: CHO 13 gm., PRO 24 gm., FAT 8 gm., Calories 216, Sodium 391 mg. (Only ¼ cup of the 1 cup milk plus salt for dipping is used up, therefore only that amount is calculated.)

Food Exchanges per serving: 1 Bread Exchange plus 3 Lean Meat Exchanges.

Low-sodium diets: Omit salt. Use unsalted crackers. Choose a freshwater fish.

Red Snapper Creole

6 servings   1 serving: 3½ ounces cooked fish plus ½ cup sauce

2 pounds red snapper fillets
2 tablespoons margarine, melted
½ cup finely cut celery
½ cup finely diced carrots
¼ cup chopped black olives
½ cup finely cut green pepper
1 cup chopped onion
1 can (16 ounces) tomatoes, cut up
½ cup tomato sauce
2 tablespoons margarine

Thaw fish if it is frozen. Preheat oven to 350° F. (180° C.). Cut fish into 6 serving pieces. Pour 2 tablespoons melted margarine into a large baking pan and set aside. Combine celery, carrots, olives, green pepper, onions, tomatoes, and tomato sauce. Spread half of this mixture in bottom of pan. Place fish pieces on top; cover with remaining mixture. Dot with margarine. Bake 30 to 35 minutes or until fish flakes with a fork.

Nutritive values per serving: CHO 10 gm., PRO 32 gm., FAT 12 gm., Calories 280, Sodium 440 mg.

Food Exchanges per serving: 4 Lean Meat Exchanges plus 2 Vegetable Exchanges.

Low-sodium diets: Use unsalted margarine, unsalted canned tomatoes, and unsalted tomato sauce. Omit the olives if sodium restriction is 1 gram per day or less.

Hearty Halibut

6 servings   1 serving: 4 ounces

2 pounds fresh or frozen halibut steaks
¾ cup thinly sliced onions
1 can (4 ounces) sliced mushrooms, drained
¾ cup chopped fresh tomato (or canned, drained)
¼ cup chopped sweet green pepper
¼ cup minced parsley
3 tablespoons finely chopped pimiento
½ cup dry, white wine
2 tablespoons white vinegar
1 teaspoon salt
⅛ teaspoon pepper
2 tablespoons margarine
Wedges of lemon for garnish

Thaw fish if frozen. Preheat oven to 350° F. (180° C.). Prepare large baking pan with vegetable pan coating (spray or solid). Cut fish into six serving pieces. Arrange onions in bottom of baking pan. Place fish on top of onions. Combine remaining ingredients except margarine and lemon wedges. Spread on top of fish. Dot with margarine. Bake 25 to 30 minutes or until fish flakes easily with a fork. Serve with lemon wedges.

Nutritive values per serving: CHO 6 gm., PRO 33 gm., FAT 6 gm., Calories 225, Sodium 1091 mg.

Food Exchanges per serving: 4 Lean Meat Exchanges plus 1 Vegetable Exchange. One Fat Exchange may be used elsewhere in the same meal because this recipe is **very** low in fat.

Low-sodium diets: This recipe is not suitable unless you substitute a freshwater fish for the halibut. Of course you will also omit the salt. Use unsalted canned mushrooms and unsalted margarine.

Cod Southwestern Style

6 servings

1 serving: 4 ounces
cooked fish
plus ⅓ cup sauce

FISH
2 pounds fresh or frozen cod fillets (use other fish fillets if preferred)
¼ teaspoon salt
⅛ teaspoon pepper
⅔ cup white wine
⅔ cup chicken broth

SAUCE
4 tablespoons margarine
½ cup chopped onions
1⅓ cup diced sweet green pepper
3 large tomatoes, peeled and diced
2 tablespoons lemon juice
1 teaspoon chili powder
½ teaspoon salt
⅛ teaspoon pepper
¼ teaspoon garlic powder
¼ teaspoon ground thyme
¼ teaspoon oregano
6 slices (about ½ ounce each) mozzarella cheese

Thaw fish if frozen. Preheat oven to 350°F. (180°C.). Divide cod into six equal portions. Place cod in a large frying pan, season with salt and pepper, pour wine and chicken broth over fish, and cover. Bring to a boil, turn heat low, and poach fish for 10 minutes. Meanwhile, prepare the sauce. Melt margarine; sauté onions, add the green pepper, and cook gently for 3 minutes. Add the remaining ingredients except the cheese slices; simmer for 10 minutes. Place fish on oven-proof serving platter. Cover fish entirely with sauce. Place a thin slice of cheese over each portion of fish. Place in oven for a few minutes, just long enough to melt cheese.

Nutritive values per serving: CHO 7 gm., PRO 31 gm., FAT 11 gm., Calories 284, Sodium 607 mg.

Food Exchanges per serving: 4 Lean Meat Exchanges plus 1 Vegetable Exchange.

Low-sodium diets: Omit salt. Use unsalted chicken broth and unsalted margarine.

Caspian Cod Fillets

6 servings   1 serving: 4 ounces

2 pounds fresh or frozen cod fillets (not salted)
3 tablespoons vegetable oil
½ cup chopped onions
¼ cup minced parsley
½ teaspoon Worcestershire sauce
¼ teaspoon salt
⅛ teaspoon crushed rosemary
⅛ teaspoon garlic powder or 1 clove garlic, crushed
Dash of pepper
Lemon wedges for garnish

Thaw cod fillets if frozen. Preheat oven to 350°F. (180°C.). Prepare large baking pan with vegetable pan coating (spray or solid). Cut fish into six equal serving pieces. Place in prepared pan. Combine remaining ingredients except lemon wedges; mix well. Spread on top of fish. Bake 30 to 40 minutes or until fish flakes easily with a fork. Serve with lemon wedges.

Nutritive values per serving: CHO 1 gm., PRO 27 gm., FAT 7 gm., Calories 185, Sodium 204 mg.

Food Exchanges per serving: 4 Lean Meat Exchanges. Because this is a very low-fat recipe you may add one more Fat Exchange elsewhere in the same meal.

Low-sodium diets: Omit salt.   Use low-sodium Worcestershire sauce.

Cantonese Shrimp and Green Beans

This one tastes so delicious Kay's nondiabetic taste-testers asked for more.

6 servings (yield: 4 cups)   1 serving: ⅔ cup

1½ pounds frozen, large, raw shrimp, deveined
1½ teaspoons instant chicken bouillon
1¼ cups boiling water
3 tablespoons vegetable oil
¼ cup slant-sliced green onions
1 clove garlic, peeled and crushed or ⅛ teaspoon garlic powder
1 teaspoon salt
½ teaspoon ground ginger or ½ teaspoon minced fresh ginger
Dash of pepper
1 package (9 ounces) frozen, cut green beans
1 tablespoon cornstarch
1 tablespoon cold water

Thaw frozen shrimp. Dissolve instant chicken bouillon in boiling water. Heat oil in a deep skillet. Cook onions, garlic, and shrimp in hot oil over medium heat for 3 minutes, stirring frequently. Stir in salt, ginger, pepper, green beans, and chicken broth; stir to mix well, then cover. Let simmer for 5 to 8 minutes until beans are crisp cooked. Stir cornstarch into cold water. Add cornstarch mixture to shrimp. Cook, stirring constantly, until thick and clear.

Nutritive values per serving: CHO 6 gm., PRO 22 gm., FAT 7 gm., Calories 187, Sodium 635 mg.

Food Exchanges per serving: 3 Lean Meat Exchanges plus 1 Vegetable Exchange. If served on ⅓ cup hot cooked rice, add 1 Bread Exchange, CHO 15 gm., PRO 2 gm., Calories 68.

Low-sodium diets: This recipe is not suitable.

Shrimp Creole

6 servings (yield: 4½ cups)   1 serving: ¾ cup

3 cups Creole Gumbo Sauce (*see* Index)
1 pound ready-to-cook fresh or frozen shrimp, deveined and without shells

Make sauce as directed in recipe. Add shrimp; bring to a boil, stirring with a wooden spoon frequently to separate shrimp. When boiling point is reached, turn heat to medium low, cover, and let simmer gently for 10 minutes; stir occasionally.

Nutritive values per serving: CHO 10 gm., PRO 16 gm., FAT 5 gm., Calories 152, Sodium 960 mg.

Food Exchanges per serving: 2 Lean Meat Exchanges plus 2 Vegetable Exchanges. If you serve this on rice, add 1 Bread Exchange, which is 68 calories, and CHO 15 gm., PRO 2 gm., for each ⅓ cup hot cooked rice.

Low-sodium diets: This recipe is not suitable.

Salmon Loaf

Canned mackerel may be used in place of salmon in this recipe to make a very good budget fish loaf.

4 servings   1 serving: ¼ loaf

1 can (16 ounces) salmon*
1 tablespoon vinegar or lemon juice
Cold water
2 medium eggs, beaten
½ teaspoon salt
⅛ teaspoon black pepper
1 slice fresh bread, finely crumbled
¼ cup finely cut celery and leaves
2 tablespoons finely cut green onions
1 tablespoon finely cut green pepper

Preheat oven to 350° F. (180° C.). Prepare a 7½-by-2¼-inch loaf pan with vegetable pan coating (spray or solid). Drain salmon, saving liquid. Discard skin but save bones. Flake salmon lightly but well with a fork (yield will be 3 cups). Crush bones (a free calcium bonus) and mix with salmon. Add vinegar to salmon liquid and add enough cold water to make ½ cup total liquid; add to salmon. Add all remaining ingredients and mix thoroughly. Pack into the prepared loaf pan. Bake 1 hour. Leave loaf in pan for 5 minutes before unmolding onto a serving plate. To serve, cut across width in 4 thick or 8 thin slices.

Nutritive values per serving: CHO 5 gm., PRO 27 gm., FAT 13 gm., Calories 253, Sodium 930 mg.

Food Exchanges per serving: 4 Lean Meat Exchanges plus 1 Vegetable Exchange.

Low-sodium diets: This recipe is not suitable.

* Canned pink and chum salmon are less expensive and as nutritious as sockeye, coho, or red salmon.

Herb Seasoning for Fish

4 servings   1 serving: 2 tablespoons

1 tablespoon finely chopped onion
1½ teaspoons dried parsley flakes or 1 tablespoon snipped, fresh parsley
1 tablespoon Worcestershire sauce
½ teaspoon salt
¼ teaspoon crushed rosemary
Dash of pepper
4 teaspoons melted margarine

Combine all ingredients. Spread over fillets. Use regular method for baking or broiling fish.

Nutritive values per serving: CHO 1 gm., PRO 0, FAT 4 gm., Calories 43, Sodium 470 mg.

Food Exchange per serving: 1 Fat Exchange.

Low-sodium diets: Omit salt. Use low-sodium Worcestershire sauce and unsalted margarine.

Sunshine Sauce

4 servings (yield: ½ cup)   1 serving: 2 tablespoons

½ cup unsweetened orange juice
1 tablespoon margarine
½ teaspoon salt
Dash of nutmeg
1 tablespoon fresh, minced parsley

Combine all ingredients in small pan. Heat until warmed through. Serve over poached or broiled fillets.

Nutritive values per serving: CHO 3 gm., PRO 0, FAT 3 gm., Calories 40, Sodium 302 mg.

Food Exchanges per serving: ½ Fruit Exchange plus ½ Fat Exchange.

Low-sodium diets: Omit salt. Use unsalted margarine.

31

Eggs, Cheese, and Yogurt

Classic French Omelet

This omelet is best made in a small nonstick frying pan or an 8-inch omelet pan. It may be served plain or filled with cheese or a vegetable mixture. Especially tasty omelets include Ratatoille omelets and Sweet Pepper omelets.

1 serving   1 serving: 1 omelet

2 large eggs
2 tablespoons water
¼ teaspoon salt
Dash pepper
2 teaspoons margarine

Mix eggs, water, salt, and pepper with a fork. Heat margarine in a skillet until hot enough to sizzle a drop of water. Reduce heat to medium. Pour in egg mixture; allow edges to set and lift mixture at edges with pancake turner to allow egg liquid to flow under the center. Slide pan back and forth over heat to keep omelet in motion so that it does not stick. When bottom is set and top is still moist, fill if desired, or turn omelet in half and slide out onto a heated plate to serve.

Nutritive values per serving: CHO 1 gm., PRO 13 gm., FAT 19 gm., Calories 232, Sodium 747 mg.

Food Exchanges per serving: 2 Medium-Fat Meat Exchanges plus 2 Fat Exchanges.

Low-sodium diets: Omit salt. Use unsalted margarine.

Puffy Omelet

Kay's friend, the late Kathryn Bele Niles, was a cookbook author and the all-time expert on cooking eggs and poultry. Kay says Mrs. Niles always recommended a 10-inch pan for a 4-egg omelet "to give it room to puff up and not over." The following was adapted from one of Mrs. Niles' basic recipes. Have eggs at room temperature before beating.

2 servings   1 serving: ½ omelet

4 large eggs, separated
½ teaspoon salt
3 tablespoons cold water
⅛ teaspoon finely ground black pepper
Dash of paprika
1 tablespoon of margarine

Preheat oven to 325° F. (165° C.). Place egg whites in a 1-quart mixing bowl. Add salt and cold water. Beat until high peaks form but whites are still bright and shiny. Add pepper and paprika to egg yolks; beat until thick, lemon colored and well mixed. Fold carefully but thoroughly into egg whites. Heat margarine in a 10-inch skillet over moderate heat until hot enough to sizzle a few drops of water. Pour in egg mixture, turn heat to low. With flat side of spatula, gently even off top surface of egg mixture. Cook slowly about 5 minutes, until evenly puffed and lightly browned on bottom. To peek at bottom, carefully lift omelet at edge with tip of spatula. Place in oven and bake about 12 to 14 minutes or until a knife tip inserted in center comes out clean. Serve immediately on warmed plates. To divide, use 2 forks and tear gently into pie-shaped pieces. Invert omelet on plates so browned bottom is on top. If desired, fold over before serving.

Nutritive values per serving: CHO 1 gm., PRO 14 gm., FAT 17 gm., Calories 215, Sodium 725 mg.

Food Exchanges per serving: 2 High-Fat Meat Exchanges.

Low-sodium diets: Omit salt. Use unsalted margarine.

Scrambled Egg Whites

Cholesterol-free scrambled eggs!

1 serving

2 tablespoons skim milk
2 egg whites
Pinch of salt
Few grains pepper
Few specks crushed marjoram
Few specks crushed thyme
1 to 2 drops yellow food color
½ teaspoon minced parsley
½ teaspoon minced onion
½ teaspoon margarine

Combine all ingredients except for margarine and mix well. Beat gently with a fork until foamy and very well blended. Melt margarine in a small frying pan to coat bottom. Add beaten egg whites. Scramble as usual over low heat.

Nutritive values per serving:　　CHO 2 gm., PRO 8 gm., FAT 2.5 gm., Calories 65, Sodium 234 mg.

Food Exchange per serving:　　1 Lean Meat Exchange.

Low-sodium diets:　　Omit salt. Use salt substitute if the doctor allows.

Never-Fail Blintzes

15 blintzes　　　　　　　　　　1 serving: 3 small, filled blintzes

FILLING
1 pound dry cottage cheese (or farmer's cheese)
1 medium egg, beaten
1 tablespoon margarine
Artificial sweetener to substitute for 1 tablespoon sugar
Dash of salt

BATTER
2 eggs, beaten until light and foamy
½ teaspoon salt
1 teaspoon sugar (needed for proper browning)
1¼ cups water
½ teaspoon grated orange rind
2 tablespoons margarine, melted
¼ teaspoon baking powder
1 cup sifted flour

To make the filling: press cheese through a ricer or fine strainer; mix well with remaining filling ingredients; set aside.

To prepare the blintzes: preheat oven to 400° F. (205° C.). Prepare a 7-inch frying pan and a shallow baking pan with vegetable pan coating (spray or solid). To make the batter, combine eggs, salt, sugar, water, orange rind, 1 tablespoon melted margarine, baking powder, and flour; beat until smooth. Pour 2½ tablespoonfuls at a time into a heated, prepared frying pan. Tip pan so batter spreads thinly over entire pan. Pour off excess. Cook over low to medium heat until top is dry and starts to blister. Turn out onto board. Put 1 tablespoon of filling on the blintz, fold in the sides, and roll until filling is enclosed. Place them in the prepared baking pan. When all blintzes are in the pan, brush tops with remaining 1 tablespoon melted margarine. Bake for 30 minutes until lightly browned.

Nutritive values per serving: CHO 21 gm., PRO 21 gm., FAT 10 gm., Calories 263, Sodium 412 mg.

Food Exchanges per serving: 2 Medium-Fat Meat Exchanges plus 1 Bread Exchange plus 1 Vegetable Exchange.

Low-sodium diets: Omit salt. Use low-sodium baking powder and unsalted margarine.

Cheese and Onion Pie

A real treat for lunch or brunch!

6 servings (yield: 9-inch pie)   1 serving: 1/6 pie

CRUST

1¼ cups soda cracker crumbs (20 crackers, crushed)
¼ cup melted margarine

FILLING

2 tablespoons margarine
2½ cups thinly sliced onions
3 medium eggs, beaten
½ cup instant nonfat dry milk powder
⅔ cup water
6 ounces Swiss cheese, shredded
¼ teaspoon salt
Dash of pepper
Dash of nutmeg

To make the crust: prepare a 9-inch pie plate with vegetable pan coating (spray or solid). Combine crumbs and margarine thoroughly; press evenly with the back of a spoon into the bottom and sides of prepared pie plate. Set aside.

To prepare the filling: preheat oven to 325° F. (165° C.). Melt margarine in a frying pan. Add onions and sauté over low heat, stirring until clear and tender but not brown. Turn onions into cracker crust and spread evenly. Combine all remaining filling ingredients and mix well. Heat over low heat, stirring only until cheese melts. Pour carefully on top of onions. Bake about 45 minutes or until custard is set. Knife tip inserted in center should come out clean.

Nutritive values per serving: CHO 17 gm., PRO 14 gm., FAT 24 gm., Calories 339, Sodium 642 mg.

Food Exchanges per serving: 1 Bread Exchange plus 2 High-Fat Meat Exchanges plus 2 Fat Exchanges.

Low-sodium diets: This recipe is not suitable.

Baked Eggs-in-Baskets

4 servings

1 serving: 1 egg in bun

4 small hamburger buns, unsliced
1 cup (4 ounces) grated American cheese
4 teaspoons catsup
4 medium eggs
Pinch of salt
Dash of pepper
2 tablespoons finely cut green onions
2 tablespoons light cream

Preheat oven to 375° F. (190° C.). Cut thin slice off top of each bun. With a fork, lift out most of the white bread and crumbs from centers of buns and discard, leaving "baskets" ½-inch thick (about 20 grams each). Place the baskets in a shallow baking pan. Spoon 2 tablespoons grated cheese into each shell; top each with 1 teaspoon catsup. One at a time, break eggs into a saucer, then slide an egg carefully into each basket. Sprinkle each lightly with salt and pepper, and the remaining grated cheese; top each with onions and cream. Bake 20 to 25 minutes or until eggs are firm.

Nutritive values per serving: CHO 13 gm., PRO 14 gm., FAT 16 gm., Calories 256, Sodium 552 mg.

Food Exchanges per serving: 2 High-Fat Meat Exchanges plus 1 Bread Exchange.

Low-sodium diets: Omit salt. Use low-sodium cheese.

Eggs Benedict

Mary's daughter Leslie, age 5, always wants this served when her kindergarten friends come for lunch. It's her favorite! The timing in making this takes a bit of practice to get the eggs poached, the muffins toasted, and the bacon and sauce all hot at the same time. Get all ingredients measured and pans ready before you start. You will need a large frying pan for the bacon, a toaster or broiler for the muffins, and a suitable pan of simmering water for poaching the eggs. Ready?

3 or 6 servings

1 serving: 2 muffin halves plus 2 eggs plus 2 bacon slices plus 4 tablespoons sauce *or,* for a small serving, 1 muffin half plus 1 egg plus 1 bacon slice plus 2 tablespoons sauce

¾ cup Mock Hollandaise Sauce (*see* Index)
3 English muffins, split
6 medium eggs
6 slices (1 ounce each) Canadian-style bacon
Parsley for garnish

Prepare the Mock Hollandaise Sauce, set aside, and cover to keep hot. Now, all at the same time, toast the split muffins, poach the eggs in simmering water, and grill bacon in a separate frying pan with no added fat. Place toasted muffin halves split side up on a plate; top each with 1 slice bacon, then a poached egg, and, finally, 2 tablespoons Mock Hollandaise Sauce. Garnish with parsley. For one large serving, serve 2 muffin halves. For one small serving, serve 1 muffin half.

Nutritive values per serving:
1 large serving— CHO 32 gm., PRO 30 gm., FAT 21
(2 muffin halves) gm., Calories 451, Sodium 1654 mg.
1 small serving— CHO 16 gm., PRO 15 gm., FAT 10
(1 muffin half) gm., Calories 225, Sodium 827 mg.

Food Exchanges per serving:
1 large serving— 2 Bread Exchanges plus 4
(2 muffin halves) Medium-Fat Meat Exchanges.
1 small serving— 1 Bread Exchange plus 2
(1 muffin half) Medium-Fat Meat Exchanges.

Low-sodium diets: This recipe is not suitable.

Baked Welsh Rarebit

4 servings   1 serving: 1 slice bread plus cheese sauce

4 slices white bread
8 slices (1 ounce each) American cheese
2 large eggs, beaten
2 tablespoons prepared mustard
1 cup skim milk
1 teaspoon salt
1 teaspoon Worcestershire sauce
Paprika or parsley for garnish

Preheat oven to 350° F. (180° C.). Place bread slices in a large, shallow casserole or oblong baking pan; do not overlap slices. Place 2 slices cheese on each slice of bread. Combine remaining ingredients; mix well. Pour on top of cheese and bread. Bake 25 minutes. Garnish with paprika or minced parsley, whichever is preferred.

Nutritive values per serving: CHO 19 gm., PRO 21 gm., FAT 21 gm., Calories 356, Sodium 1526 mg.

Food Exchanges per serving: 1 Bread Exchange plus 3 High-Fat Meat Exchanges.

Low-sodium diets: This recipe is not suitable.

Apple Pancake

A great brunch or luncheon entree.

4 servings   1 serving: ¼ pancake

CINNAMON TOPPING
1 teaspoon ground cinnamon
Artificial sweetener to substitute for ¼ cup sugar

PANCAKE
1 large (300 grams) cooking apple
½ cup skim milk
½ cup flour
3 medium eggs, beaten
1 teaspoon sugar (needed for browning)
Dash of salt
2 tablespoons margarine
2 tablespoons lemon juice

Preheat oven to 400° F. (205° C.). For cinnamon mixture, combine cinnamon and artificial sweetener, and mix well; set aside. Cut apple in very thin slices, removing core. Combine the skim milk, flour, eggs, sugar, and salt, and mix until smooth; do not beat. Melt 1 tablespoon of the margarine in a 10-inch frying pan and "roll" it around so sides and bottom are covered. Add sliced apples and sauté slightly. Pour batter on top evenly. Bake in oven about 10 minutes or until pancake is puffy and nearly cooked. Sprinkle top with cinnamon mixture, dot with remaining 1 tablespoon margarine, return to oven to brown pancake. Before serving, sprinkle with lemon juice. Cut in quarters to serve.

Nutritive values per serving: CHO 25 gm., PRO 7 gm., FAT 10 gm., Calories 219, Sodium 160 mg.

Food Exchanges per serving: 1 Bread Exchange plus 1 Fruit Exchange plus 1 High-Fat Meat Exchange.

Low-sodium diets: Omit salt. Use unsalted margarine.

Orange French Toast

2 or 4 servings

1 serving: 1 to 2 slices toast, excluding sweet spread

2 medium eggs, beaten very lightly
⅓ cup unsweetened orange juice or the juice of 1 medium orange
½ teaspoon pure vanilla
1 teaspoon grated orange peel
4 slices bread (day-old bread is better than fresh)
2 teaspoons margarine

Mix together the eggs, orange juice, vanilla, and orange peel; pour into a pie plate. Dip each slice of bread into mixture until all liquid is absorbed into bread. Heat margarine in a large frying pan over medium heat and lightly brown bread on both sides. Serve warm with one of the sweet spreads (*see* Index).

Nutritive values per serving:

1 slice—
CHO 16 gm., PRO 5 gm., FAT 5 gm., Calories 138, Sodium 192 mg.

2 slices—
CHO 33 gm., PRO 11 gm., FAT 11 gm., Calories 277, Sodium 384 mg.

Food Exchanges per serving:

1 slice—
1 Bread Exchange plus ½ High-Fat Meat Exchange.

2 slices—
2 Bread Exchanges plus 1 Medium-Fat Meat Exchange plus 1 Fat Exchange.

Low-sodium diets:
Use low-sodium bread and unsalted margarine.

Blueberry Yogurt

2 servings (yield: 1⅓ cups)   1 serving: ⅔ cup

½ cup (75 grams) blueberries
Artificial sweetener to substitute for 1 tablespoon sugar
¼ teaspoon vanilla extract
1 cup plain, low-fat yogurt

Wash blueberries; mash them with artificial sweetener. Stir vanilla into yogurt; fold in blueberries. Chill in a small covered container for several hours or overnight.

Nutritive values per serving: CHO 11 gm., PRO 4 gm., FAT 2 gm., Calories 79, Sodium 58 mg.

Food Exchanges per serving: ½ Milk Exchange plus ½ Fruit Exchange plus ½ Fat Exchange.

Low-sodium diets: This recipe is suitable.

Peach Yogurt

2 servings (yield: 1⅓ cups)   1 serving: ⅔ cup

⅔ cup (125 grams) fresh peaches, pared and diced
½ teaspoon lemon juice
Artificial sweetener to substitute for 1 tablespoon sugar
1 cup plain, low-fat yogurt

Slightly mash diced peaches with lemon juice and sweetener. Stir in yogurt; blend well. Chill in a covered container several hours or overnight.

Nutritive values per serving: CHO 12 gm., PRO 4 gm., FAT 2 gm., Calories 80, Sodium 58 mg.

Food Exchanges per serving: ½ Milk Exchange plus ½ Fruit Exchange plus ½ Fat Exchange.

Low-sodium diets: This recipe is suitable.

Raspberry Yogurt

2 servings (yield: 1⅓ cups)   1 serving: ⅔ cup

½ cup fresh raspberries
Artificial sweetener to substitute for 1 tablespoon sugar
1 cup plain, low-fat yogurt

Wash raspberries; mash them with the sweetener. Stir in yogurt and mix well. Chill in a covered container several hours or overnight.

Nutritive values per serving: CHO 10 gm., PRO 4 gm., FAT 2 gm., Calories 74, Sodium 58 mg.

Food Exchanges per serving: ½ Milk Exchange plus ½ Fruit Exchange plus ½ Fat Exchange.

Low-sodium diets: This recipe is suitable.

Strawberry Yogurt

2 servings (yield: 1⅓ cups)   1 serving: ⅔ cup

¾ cup whole strawberries
1 teaspoon lemon juice
Artificial sweetener to substitute for 1 tablespoon sugar
1 cup plain, low-fat yogurt

Wash and hull strawberries; cut them into small pieces. Add lemon juice and sweetener; mix well. Combine with yogurt; mix thoroughly. Chill in a small covered container for several hours or overnight.

Nutritive values per serving: CHO 11 gm., PRO 4 gm., FAT 2 gm., Calories 77, Sodium 58 mg.

Food Exchanges per serving: ½ Milk Exchange plus ½ Fruit Exchange plus ½ Fat Exchange.

Low-sodium diets: This recipe is suitable.

32

Potatoes, Pasta, and Rice

Roasted Potatoes

This is also lovely made with small new red potatoes. If you use these do not peel the potatoes. The skins are tender and delicious.

4 servings   1 serving: 2 pieces of potato

1 pound (about 2 medium) potatoes
Boiling water
1 teaspoon salt, for the cooking water
2 tablespoons margarine, melted
½ teaspoon salt
⅛ teaspoon pepper
1 tablespoon finely minced fresh parsley

Prepare a pie plate with vegetable pan coating (spray or solid). Wash potatoes; boil them in their skins in salted boiling water to cover for 20 to 25 minutes or until tender when pierced with a fork. Preheat oven to 400° F. (205° C.). Drain potatoes and peel them immediately. Cut each potato in four pieces and place potatoes on prepared pie plate; baste each potato with melted margarine, sprinkle with salt, pepper, and parsley. Roast in oven 15 minutes until potatoes are nicely browned.

Nutritive values per serving: CHO 15 gm., PRO 2 gm., FAT 2 gm., Calories 82, Sodium 559 mg.

Food Exchange per serving: 1 Bread Exchange plus ½ Fat Exchange.

Low-sodium diets: Omit salt. Use unsalted margarine.

Baked "French Fries'

5 servings (yield: 50 to 60 pieces)   1 serving: 10 to 12 pieces

2 large (500 grams) potatoes
1 tablespoon vegetable oil
½ teaspoon salt
⅛ teaspoon paprika

Preheat oven to 450° F. (230° C.). Peel potatoes, cut into slices 4 inches long and ¼ inch wide; place in a bowl of iced water to crisp. Just before cooking turn onto paper towels and pat dry. Spread pieces in one layer on a shallow baking pan. Sprinkle with the vegetable oil. Shake pan to spread oil evenly over potatoes. Bake 30 to 40 minutes, turning frequently, until golden brown. Empty potatoes onto paper towels. Sprinkle with salt and paprika.

Nutritive values per serving: CHO 15 gm., PRO 2 gm., FAT 2 gm., Calories 82, Sodium 110 mg.

Food Exchanges per serving: 1 Bread Exchange plus ½ Fat Exchange.

Low-sodium diets: Omit salt.   Use a seasoned salt substitute, if allowed by your doctor.

Scalloped Potatoes

5 servings (yield: 2½ cups)   1 serving: ½ cup

1 pound potatoes
2 tablespoons flour
½ teaspoon salt
⅛ teaspoon pepper
2 tablespoons margarine
3 tablespoons finely chopped onion
Hot water

Preheat oven to 400° F. (205° C.). Prepare a 1½-quart casserole with vegetable pan coating (spray or solid). Pare potatoes; slice potatoes crosswise in ⅛-inch slices; if potatoes are large, cut slices in half. Mix together flour, salt, and pepper. Place half of potatoes in prepared casserole. Dot with half the margarine, sprinkle half the seasoned flour on top, then half the onions. Repeat with remaining potatoes, margarine, seasoned flour, and onions. Pour enough hot water in, at one corner only, so that the water barely comes to the top of the potatoes. Cover and bake 50 minutes; then uncover and bake for another 25 to 30 minutes or until potatoes are browned and tender.

Nutritive values per serving: CHO 16 gm., PRO 2 gm., FAT 5 gm., Calories 111, Sodium 272 mg.

Food Exchanges per serving: 1 Bread Exchange plus 1 Fat Exchange.

Low-sodium diets: Omit salt. Use unsalted margarine.

Giant Potato Pancake

Use Idaho potatoes in this recipe because they are more solid and grate better than most other varieties. The turning is tricky!

6 servings   1 serving: ⅙ pancake

1½ pounds Idaho potatoes
¼ cup finely chopped onion
1 teaspoon salt
¼ teaspoon pepper
1 tablespoon margarine

Pare potatoes with a vegetable peeler. Grate potatoes on medium grater into a large bowl. Add onion, salt, and pepper, and mix lightly but well with a blending fork. Melt margarine in a 10-inch frying pan and rotate to coat bottom and sides of pan. Turn potatoes into pan; pat down and spread evenly. Cover pan tightly; turn heat low and let cook about 15 minutes or until underside is browned. Take pan off heat temporarily. Put a 12-inch plate (or very large pie plate) upside down on top of potatoes and, with one hand on handle of frying pan and the other hand guiding the plate, turn frying pan upside down, then lift off of the pancake. This puts the pancake on the plate. Next, immediately slide pancake back into the frying pan, browned side up. Return to slow heat. Do not cover. Let cook for another 15 minutes or until bottom is browned. To serve, cut evenly into 6 pie-shaped wedges.

Nutritive values per serving: CHO 18 gm., PRO 2 gm., FAT 2 gm., Calories 97, Sodium 382 mg.

Food Exchanges per serving: 1 Bread Exchange plus ½ Fat Exchange.

Low-sodium diets: Omit salt. Use unsalted margarine.

Pratie Cakes

Certain Irish folk refer to potato cakes as "praties." They are great! Mix and shape ahead, then chill before cooking.

7 servings (yield: 7 cakes)   1 serving: a 3-inch cake

2 cups cold, mashed potatoes (fresh or prepared from flakes)
½ cup unsifted flour (reserve 1 tablespoon for flouring board)
¼ teaspoon salt
2 tablespoons finely chopped onions
2 tablespoons margarine

Turn mashed potatoes into a large bowl. Add flour, salt, and onions. Mix thoroughly with hands and fingers, until completely mixed and smooth. Pat on a lightly floured board until ½ inch thick. Cut with a 3-inch floured cookie cutter. Place on a cookie sheet, cover lightly with waxed paper, chill in refrigerator until just before cooking. To cook, use 1 tablespoon margarine at a time. Melt margarine in a large frying pan or stove-top griddle. Fry cakes over moderately hot heat, turning to brown on both sides. Serve immediately.

Nutritive values per serving: CHO 15 gm., PRO 2 gm., FAT 4 gm., Calories 103, Sodium 297 mg.

Food Exchanges per serving: 1 Bread Exchange plus 1 Fat Exchange.

Low-sodium diets: Omit salt from original mashed potato mixture and from recipe. Use unsalted margarine.

German Potato Salad

8 servings (yield: 4 cups)   1 serving: ½ cup

4 medium-sized potatoes (about 1½ pounds)
½ teaspoon salt, for cooking potatoes
4 medium slices bacon
¾ cup chopped onion
¾ cup chopped celery
¾ cup water
¼ cup cider vinegar
1 tablespoon flour
1½ tablespoons sugar
½ teaspoon salt
¼ teaspoon pepper
1 tablespoon fresh minced parsley

Pare and cook potatoes in boiling salted water to cover until tender, about 25 minutes. Meanwhile, fry bacon in a large frying pan over low heat until crisp. Lift bacon out of fat and place on paper towel. To bacon fat in the frying pan add onions and celery; cook and stir over medium heat until onions are slightly browned. Add remaining ingredients except parsley, potatoes, and bacon, to the frying pan and cook, stirring, about 10 minutes until sauce is thick and smooth. Drain potatoes and slice them in thin rounds. Add potatoes to frying pan and toss with hot sauce. Chop bacon strips and toss bacon bits and chopped parsley into potatoes. Serve this potato salad warm.

Nutritive values per serving: CHO 16 gm., PRO 3 gm., FAT 9 gm., Calories 154, Sodium 303 mg.

Food Exchanges per serving: 1 Bread Exchange plus 2 Fat Exchanges.

Low-sodium diets: This recipe is not suitable.

Zesty Potato Salad

6 servings (yield: almost 4 cups)   1 serving: ⅔ cup

2½ cups diced cooked potatoes
½ cup finely chopped onion
¼ cup chopped parsley
¼ cup finely cut celery
½ cup plain, low-fat yogurt
1 tablespoon prepared mustard
¾ teaspoon herb or Italian seasoning
1 hard-cooked egg, sliced
¼ teaspoon paprika

Combine the potatoes, onions, parsley, and celery; then mix. In a small bowl combine the yogurt, mustard, and seasoning; add to vegetables; mix carefully. Cover and chill several hours to allow flavors to blend. When serving, garnish with slices of egg and paprika.

Nutritive values per serving: CHO 12 gm., PRO 3 gm., FAT 1 gm., Calories 74, Sodium 76 mg.

Food Exchange per serving: 1 Bread Exchange.

Low-sodium diets: This recipe is suitable.

Boiled Sweet Potatoes

Because sweet potatoes are high in carbohydrates, only ¼ cup of mashed, cooked sweet potatoes yields 17 grams CHO, which may be counted as 1 Bread Exchange. So, let's be on guard and not be greedy!

5 servings (yield: 2 cups)   1 serving: for the diabetic serve ¼ cup

1½ pounds sweet potatoes
Boiling water
1½ tablespoons margarine, cut in pieces
¼ teaspoon pumpkin pie spice mixture

Scrub potatoes thoroughly; cut off and discard small ends and inedible knobs. If potatoes are large, cut in halves or thirds. Place in a deep cooking pot, then cover with boiling water. Cover pot, bring to a boil, and cook over moderate heat until potatoes are soft (about 25 minutes). Drain at once. Hold each potato with a fork and peel quickly. Place potatoes in a bowl, mash and beat with margarine and pumpkin pie spice.

Nutritive values per ¼ cup
    serving: CHO 17 gm., PRO 1 gm., FAT 3 gm., Calories 99, Sodium 33 mg.

Food Exchanges per ¼ cup
    serving: 1 Bread Exchange plus ½ Fat Exchange.

Low-sodium diets: Use unsalted margarine.

Mary's Macaroni Salad

7 servings (yield: 3½ cups)   1 serving: ½ cup

3 cups (390 grams) hot macaroni, drained, cooked firm
⅓ cup Low-Calorie Cooked Dressing (*see* Index)
⅓ cup thinly sliced celery
2 tablespoons finely minced fresh parsley
1 tablespoon chopped green onion, with tops
2 hard-cooked eggs, sliced
½ teaspoon salt
¼ teaspoon coarsely ground pepper

Mix all ingredients together in a large bowl while macaroni is hot. Cover and chill in the refrigerator several hours before serving.

Nutritive values per serving: CHO 18 gm., PRO 5 gm., FAT 2 gm., Calories 113, Sodium 330 mg.

Food Exchanges per serving: 1 Bread Exchange plus ½ Medium-Fat Meat Exchange.

Low-sodium diets: Omit salt in cooking water for macaroni and in this recipe. Omit salt in Low-Calorie Cooked Dressing recipe.

Pasta Primavera

A typical Italian preparation of pasta without a hint of tomato sauce. It is scrumptious hot, but may also be served at room temperature as a pasta salad for a buffet or picnic.

6 servings (yield: 6¼ cups)   1 serving: 1 cup *or*, for
                                     a small serving, ½ cup

½ pound box of thin spaghetti,
  cooked according to package directions
½ pound broccoli*
2 tablespoons olive oil
2 cloves garlic, peeled and crushed
½ pound young zucchini,* washed and thinly sliced
½ pound mushrooms, sliced
1½ teaspoons dried basil
½ teaspoon salt
½ teaspoon coarsely ground pepper
2 tablespoons water
2 tablespoons grated Parmesan cheese

While spaghetti is cooking, wash broccoli and cook it in a small amount of boiling water until crisp but tender. Meanwhile, heat 1 tablespoon olive oil in a large frying pan and sauté garlic 3 minutes; add zucchini and cook until slightly browned. Add mushrooms; cook until mushrooms are tender. Drain broccoli; slice into bite-sized pieces and add it to zucchini and mushrooms. Stir in seasonings. When spaghetti is "al dente" stop cooking by pouring cold water into pot; drain spaghetti. Return it to the pot, stir in 2 tablespoons of water, remaining 1 tablespoon olive oil, Parmesan cheese, and vegetable mixture. Cover and reheat over low heat.

Nutritive values per serving:
    1 cup—   CHO 35 gm., PRO 8 gm., FAT 6
                        gm., Calories 223, Sodium 367 mg.
    ½ cup—   CHO 18 gm., PRO 4 gm., FAT 3
                        gm., Calories 112, Sodium 184 mg.

  * You may substitute eggplant, red or green sweet peppers, green beans, onions or other vegetables in season.

Food Exchanges per serving:

1 cup—	2 Bread Exchanges plus 1 Vegetable Exchange plus 1 Fat Exchange.
½ cup—	1 Bread Exchange plus ½ Vegetable Exchange plus ½ Fat Exchange.

Low-sodium diets: Omit salt in recipe and in cooking water of spaghetti.

Beef-Flavored Pilaf

4 servings (yield: 2 cups)   1 serving: ½ cup

2 teaspoons vegetable oil
½ cup raw rice
¼ cup finely chopped onion
1 cup beef broth
¼ cup water
2 tablespoons snipped parsley

Combine oil, raw rice, and onions into a 1½-quart saucepan. Stir over medium heat with a wooden spoon until rice is lightly browned. Add broth and water; bring to boil. Cover and simmer 20 minutes or until rice is tender and liquid is absorbed. Stir occasionally with a fork and use a lifting motion to prevent rice kernels from lumping. Just before serving use a fork to gently mix in the parsley.

Nutritive values per serving: CHO 21 gm., PRO 3 gm., FAT 2 gm., Calories 120, Sodium 198 mg.

Food Exchanges per serving: 1½ Bread Exchanges. (A ⅓ cup serving is equal to 1 Bread Exchange.)

Low-sodium diets: Use low-sodium beef bouillon cube dissolved in 1¼ cups water and omit the broth and water in the recipe.

Curried Rice

6 servings (yield: 3 cups)   1 serving: ½ cup *or,* for a
                                              small serving, ⅓ cup

2½ cups cold water
3 chicken bouillon cubes
1 cup raw rice
1½ teaspoons margarine
1 teaspoon curry powder

Combine all ingredients in a heavy saucepan. Bring to a boil, stirring with a fork until bouillon cubes are dissolved. Cover tightly, reduce heat to simmer, and cook 15 to 20 minutes. Turn heat off, remove lid, and let pan stand 2 to 3 minutes; stirring occasionally with a fork until rice is fluffy and dry.

Nutritive values per serving:
    ½ cup—   CHO 26 gm., PRO 3 gm., FAT 1 gm., Calories 129, Sodium 493 mg.
    ⅓ cup—   CHO 17 gm., PRO 1 gm., FAT 1 gm., Calories 82, Sodium 329 mg.

Food Exchanges per serving:
    ½ cup—   1½ Bread Exchanges.
    ⅓ cup—   1 Bread Exchange.

Low-sodium diets: Use low-sodium chicken bouillon cubes and unsalted margarine.

Rice with Mushrooms

5 servings (yield: 3¼ cups)   1 serving: ⅔ cup *or,* for
                                           a small serving, ⅓ cup

2 cups water
2 chicken bouillon cubes
½ teaspoon salt
1 cup raw rice
1 can (4 ounces) mushroom stems and pieces
2 tablespoons margarine
⅛ teaspoon pepper
Few sprigs parsley for garnish

Bring water, bouillon cubes, and salt to a boil. Add rice slowly, stirring with a fork, and cook according to cooking time indicated on rice package. (Different types of rice vary in cooking times.) All water should be absorbed when the rice is cooked. Drain mushrooms and pour liquid from can into water with the rice. Heat margarine in a small saucepan; sauté drained mushrooms in margarine until they are slightly browned. When rice is cooked, toss mushrooms and pepper into rice and stir with a fork to mix. Serve in a bowl topped with parsley sprigs.

Nutritive values per serving:

⅔ cup—   CHO 32 gm., PRO 3 gm., FAT 5 gm., Calories 188, Sodium 735 mg.

⅓ cup—   CHO 16 gm., PRO 2 gm., FAT 2 gm., Calories 94, Sodium 368 mg.

Food Exchanges per serving:

⅔ cup—   2 Bread Exchanges plus 1 Fat Exchange.

⅓ cup—   1 Bread Exchange plus ½ Fat Exchange.

Low-sodium diets: Omit salt. Use low-sodium bouillon cubes, unsalted margarine, and unsalted canned or fresh mushrooms.

Rice Pallau

6 servings (yield: 3 cups)   1 serving: ½ cup *or*, for
                                              a small serving, ⅓ cup

1 cup raw rice
⅛ teaspoon saffron
½ teaspoon cumin seed
2 cups water
½ teaspoon salt
1 tablespoon minced, fresh parsley

Soak saffron in 2 tablespoons water (to get color). Combine in a
1½-quart cooking pot the rice, saffron, cumin seed, water, and salt.
Bring to a boil, cover, and cook over low heat about 20 minutes or
until water is just absorbed. If necessary, toss lightly with a fork.
Mix parsley with rice before serving.

Nutritive values per serving:
    ½ cup—   CHO 26 gm., PRO 2 gm., FAT 0,
                                              Calories 118, Sodium 180 mg.
    ⅓ cup—   CHO 17 gm., PRO 1 gm., FAT 0,
                                              Calories 79, Sodium 120 mg.

Food Exchanges per serving:
    ½ cup—   1½ Bread Exchanges.
    ⅓ cup—   1 Bread Exchange.

Low-sodium diets: Omit salt.

Rizzi Bizzi

This is one of Mary's "specials"—try it!

6 servings (yield: 4 cups)   1 serving: ⅔ cup

1½ cups water
1 chicken bouillon cube
½ teaspoon salt
1 tablespoon margarine
¾ cup raw rice
1 package (10 ounces) frozen peas
¼ cup finely cut green onions

Bring water, chicken bouillon cube, salt, and margarine to a boil. Add rice slowly, stirring with a fork, and cook according to package directions. Cook peas according to package directions until crisp but tender. When rice is cooked, add peas and green onions; mix well. Serve with roast chicken, roast lamb, or other meats.

Nutritive values per serving: CHO 25 gm., PRO 4 gm., FAT 2 gm., Calories 137, Sodium 670 mg.

Food Exchanges per serving: 1 Bread Exchange plus 2 Vegetable Exchanges.

Low-sodium diets: Omit salt. Use low-sodium chicken bouillon cube, unsalted margarine. Omit frozen peas, and use 1 small can (8 ounces) low-sodium peas.

33

Vegetables

Great Vegetables

Vegetables that are cooked just right are a wonderful addition to meals. They are colorful, flavorful, and crunchy—and excellent sources of many vitamins and minerals. Vegetables fresh and in season are usually the tastiest as well as the most economical choice. So don't think of vegetables as just another food or something you *have* to include. Choose them and cook them to enjoy them!

American cooks are notorious for ruining vegetables by overcooking them. No food can become so unappetizing and tasteless as badly cooked vegetables.

There is an art in cooking vegetables and it is very simple:

- Any vegetable should be cooked only long enough to make it tender. Overcooking makes vegetables soft and mushy, and destroys the nutritive values as well.
- Cook strong-flavored vegetables in a large quantity of boiling water, uncovered, only long enough to make them tender. Place a

slice of stale bread on top to absorb cooking odors. The bread is discarded, so it is not included in the calculations for nutritive values and Food Exchanges.

- Cook mild-flavored vegetables (when cooked in water), in only a small amount of rapidly boiling water in a covered pan with a tight-fitting lid.

To prepare greens, such as spinach, beet tops, collards, or kale, for cooking, wash them under lots of running water. Spinach needs no additional water except that which clings to the leaves. Other greens will need the addition of a few tablespoons of water. Greens like privacy; be sure to cover the pot tightly and cook quickly.

There are four especially fine methods of vegetable cookery that we recommend. Each is used in one or more vegetable recipes in this book.

Baking or *oven-cooking* may be used for fresh, frozen, or canned vegetables or for dried vegetables prepared for cooking. Choose the right temperature, the right casserole size, and the right timing.

The *boiling* method has been covered briefly in the reference to strong-flavored and mild-flavored vegetables. We advise no more than ½- to 1-inch water in the pan. Some vegetables, such as new potatoes and sweet potatoes, take very well indeed to being boiled in their jackets. Peel the sweet potatoes immediately, but leave the tender skins on the new potatoes.

Steaming is an excellent cooking method that helps preserve the flavor and food values of vegetables. A regulation vegetable steamer basket that may be used in most pots is a handy piece of equipment. Make sure the bottom of the steamer does not touch the water, and keep the saucepan tightly covered. That way the steam will cook the vegetable in its own liquids. Steamed vegetables are so tasty they need little additional seasoning.

Sautéing may also be called *stir-frying* when applied to certain types of foods or recipes. A small amount of fat, sometimes with a small amount of liquid, is used in a large frying pan or wok. Vegetables alone, or meat and vegetables together, may be cooked over rather high heat and stirred with a wooden spoon during this quick hot cooking method. Vegetables should be hot but crisp and crunchy.

Try our vegetable recipes! Good eating!

Asparagus au Gratin

4 servings   1 serving: 4 to 6 spears

1 pound asparagus (16 to 24 spears)
¼ teaspoon vegetable oil (to oil pan)
3 tablespoons grated Parmesan cheese
3 tablespoons water
2 tablespoons chopped green onion
1 tablespoon margarine, melted
3 tablespoons fine dry bread crumbs
Dash of black pepper

Preheat oven to 350° F. (180° C.). Snap stems of asparagus at break point to remove woody ends; discard ends. Wash spears well to remove all soil under leaf tips. Arrange in a large, shallow frying pan and cover with boiling water. Cover pan, bring to a boil, and let cook briskly, about 8 to 10 minutes. Drain carefully. Arrange half of the spears in a single layer in a lightly oiled shallow casserole or baking pan. Sprinkle with half of the cheese; add the water. Cover with remaining asparagus; sprinkle with remaining cheese. Mix together all the other ingredients with a fork, then spread on top of asparagus. Bake covered for 15 minutes.

Nutritive values per serving: CHO 7 gm., PRO 4 gm., FAT 4 gm., Calories 82, Sodium 102 mg.

Food Exchanges per serving: 1 Vegetable Exchange plus 1 Fat Exchange.

Low-sodium diets: Substitute unsalted margarine and crumble low-sodium bread to replace crumbs.

Broccoli with Lemon

Mary's children call broccoli stalks "little trees" and they love them!

8 servings (yield: 6 cups, loosely packed)   1 serving: ¾ cup

1¾ pounds broccoli
¼ teaspoon salt
2 tablespoons margarine
2 tablespoons lemon juice
½ lemon, cut in thin wedges, for garnish

Wash broccoli and trim off tough stems. Cut each stalk of broccoli into several pieces from top to bottom for more uniform cooking. Put broccoli into a vegetable steamer basket over boiling water. Sprinkle with salt; cover pan tightly. Simmer 12 to 15 minutes or until broccoli is crisp-tender. Meanwhile melt margarine; add lemon juice. Arrange broccoli in a serving dish; drizzle margarine-lemon mixture over broccoli and garnish with lemon wedges.

Nutritive values per serving: CHO 5 gm., PRO 3 gm., FAT 3 gm., Calories 53, Sodium 114 mg.

Food Exchanges per serving: 1 Vegetable Exchange plus ½ Fat Exchange.

Low-sodium diets: Omit salt. Use unsalted margarine.

Broccoli Hollandaise

Cook the broccoli in the same way but substitute Mock Hollandaise Sauce (*see* Index) for the margarine-lemon mixture.

Brussels Sprouts with Cheese Crumbs

5 servings (yield: 2½ cups, loosely packed)   1 serving: ½ cup

1 package (10 ounces) frozen Brussels sprouts
1 cup boiling water
¼ teaspoon salt
1 teaspoon lemon juice
2 tablespoons cheese cracker crumbs (10 small crackers, crushed)

Cook sprouts in boiling salted water in an uncovered pan. Simmer over medium heat 10 to 12 minutes or until tender when pierced with a fork; drain sprouts. Sprinkle with lemon juice and crumbs; mix to blend.

Nutritive values per serving: CHO 5 gm., PRO 2 gm., FAT 1 gm., Calories 30, Sodium 137 gm.

Food Exchange per serving: 1 Vegetable Exchange.

Low-sodium diets: Omit salt.

Sweet and Sour Red Cabbage

8 servings (yield: 6 cups)   1 serving: ¾ cup

1 pound red cabbage, shredded
½ cup cider vinegar
½ cup water
2 tablespoons margarine
½ teaspoon salt
Artificial sweetener to substitute for 2 tablespoons sugar

Put cabbage, vinegar, water, margarine, and salt in a deep cooking pot. Cover and cook about 15 minutes or until crisp-tender, lifting and turning with a large kitchen fork 2 or 3 times. Remove from heat. Crush artificial sweetening tablets and dissolve in a small amount of water. Add to cabbage gradually, lifting and mixing well with a fork. Drain off any liquid.

Nutritive values per serving: CHO 5 gm., PRO 1 gm., FAT 3 gm., Calories 45, Sodium 183 mg.

Food Exchanges per serving: 1 Vegetable Exchange plus ½ Fat Exchange.

Low-sodium diets: Omit salt. Use unsalted margarine.

Dilled Carrots

5 servings (yield: 2½ cups)

1 serving: ½ cup (about 7 strips)

1 pound young tender carrots, without tops
1½ tablespoons margarine
¼ teaspoon dill weed
¼ teaspoon salt
Dash pepper
1 tablespoon water

Preheat oven to 375° F. (190° C.). Pare carrots with vegetable peeler or scrub them very well with a vegetable brush. Cut carrots into strips, like French fries. Place carrots in the middle of a piece of heavy-duty foil; dot with margarine and sprinkle with seasonings and water. Wrap carrots securely in foil and crimp edges. Bake 45 minutes or until carrots are tender.

Nutritive values per serving: CHO 4 gm., PRO 1 gm., FAT 3 gm., Calories 50, Sodium 169 mg.

Food Exchanges per serving: 1 Vegetable Exchange plus ½ Fat Exchange.

Low-sodium diets: Omit salt. Use unsalted margarine.

Orange Spiced Carrots

Rachel, age 7, is our severest critic. She loved these!

4 servings (yield: 2 cups)   1 serving: ½ cup

1 pound young tender carrots, without tops
½ cup water
½ cup orange juice
1 tablespoon margarine
½ teaspoon pure vanilla
¼ teaspoon ground nutmeg
1½ teaspoons grated, fresh orange rind

Wash carrots and pare them with a vegetable peeler; remove ends. Cut carrots crosswise into ¼-inch rounds. In a saucepan put water, orange juice, and margarine; add carrots. Cover tightly and simmer over low heat 25 minutes or until carrots are crisp-tender. Check to make sure that carrots don't burn because most of the liquid will be absorbed; add a few tablespoons of water if necessary. Sprinkle carrots with vanilla, nutmeg, and orange rind; mix well.

Nutritive values per serving: CHO 9 gm., PRO 1 gm., FAT 3 gm., Calories 71, Sodium 41 mg.

Food Exchanges per serving: 1 Vegetable Exchange plus ½ Fruit Exchange plus ½ Fat Exchange.

Low-sodium diets: Use unsalted margarine.

Cauliflower Crown

6 servings   1 serving: ⅙ head (about ¾ cup)

1 small (1½ pounds) cauliflower
1 quart boiling water
1 teaspoon lemon juice
1 teaspoon salt
1 slice bread
¼ cup plain, low-fat yogurt
1 tablespoon margarine
¼ teaspoon paprika

Trim tough stem and old leaves off whole head of cauliflower, leaving tender leaves and stems. Even off the bottom. Place in a deep, cooking pot with boiling water, lemon juice, and salt. Place bread slice on top to absorb odor. Preheat oven to 350° F. (180° C.). Let cauliflower cook briskly for about 20 minutes or until cauliflower stem is fork tender. Discard bread slice. Drain cauliflower carefully but thoroughly. Place cauliflower stem side down on a foil-lined baking sheet. Put yogurt just in the center of the top of the cauliflower to form a "crown." Divide the margarine into small bits and dot margarine around yogurt. Sprinkle evenly with paprika. Bake for 10 minutes.

Nutritive values per serving.   CHO 6 gm., PRO 3 gm., FAT 2 gm., Calories 52, Sodium 100 mg. (estimated).

Food Exchanges per serving: 1 Vegetable Exchange plus ½ Fat Exchange.

Low-sodium diets: Omit salt. Use unsalted margarine.

Cauliflower in Cheese Sauce

6 servings (yield: approximately 3¾ cups)   1 serving: ⅔ cup

1 small head (1 pound) cauliflower
1 slice bread
1 teaspoon salt
1 tablespoon lemon juice
½ cup skim milk
½ cup (2 ounces) shredded Cheddar cheese
1 tablespoon margarine
1 tablespoon flour
1 tablespoon fresh chopped parsley
Dash cayenne pepper

Preheat oven to 325° F. (165° C.). Prepare a 1½-quart oven-proof casserole with vegetable pan coating. Wash cauliflower, remove leaves and core, and divide into flowerets. Put in a pot with boiling water to cover; add bread, salt, and lemon juice. Cook cauliflower over medium heat about 15 to 20 minutes until it is fork tender. Meanwhile, in the top of a double boiler, heat the milk, add the cheese, and stir to blend; add remaining ingredients and cook until cheese mixture is thick and smooth. Drain the cauliflower and discard bread; place cauliflower in the prepared casserole. Pour cheese sauce evenly over top. Bake uncovered 15 minutes.

Nutritive values per serving: CHO 6 gm., PRO 5 gm., FAT 5 gm., Calories 84, Sodium 240 mg.

Food Exchanges per serving: 1 Vegetable Exchange plus 1 Fat Exchange.

Low-sodium diets: Omit salt. Use low-sodium cheese and use unsalted margarine.

Cauliflower and Tomatoes

4 servings (yield: 2¾ cups)   1 serving: ⅔ cup

1 package (10 ounces) frozen cauliflower
2 finely cut green onions
1 tablespoon margarine
½ teaspoon salt
1 can (10 ounces) tomatoes, cut up with liquid
2 tablespoons grated American cheese

Cook cauliflower as directed on package; drain and return to saucepan. Add green onions, margarine, salt, tomatoes, and tomato liquid. Cover tightly and simmer 2 to 3 minutes. Turn into a serving dish; sprinkle cheese on top.

Nutritive values per serving: CHO 6 gm., PRO 3 gm., FAT 4 gm., Calories 68, Sodium 611 mg.

Food Exchanges per serving: 1 Vegetable Exchange plus 1 Fat Exchange.

Low-sodium diets: This recipe is not suitable.

Braised Celery and Mushrooms

4 servings (yield: 2 cups)   1 serving: ½ cup

2 cups slant-sliced celery
1 can (4 ounces) mushroom pieces, drained
¼ cup chopped onion
1 chicken bouillon cube
1 cup boiling water
½ teaspoon Worcestershire sauce

Place celery in a large frying pan. Scatter mushroom pieces and onions on top. Dissolve bouillon cube in boiling water, add Worcestershire sauce, and stir. Pour on top of vegetables. Bring to a boil, cover, reduce heat, and simmer 10 minutes or until celery is crisptender.

Nutritive values per serving: CHO 4 gm., PRO 1 gm., FAT 0, Calories 18, Sodium 441 mg.

Food Exchange per serving: 1 Vegetable Exchange.

Low-sodium diets: This recipe is not suitable.

Corn Creole

4 servings (yield: 2 cups)   1 serving: ½ cup

1 tablespoon margarine
½ cup finely chopped onion
½ cup finely chopped sweet green pepper
1 can (16 ounces) corn, drained (not cream-style)
½ cup canned tomatoes, cut up with liquid
½ teaspoon chili powder (more or less)
½ teaspoon salt
¼ teaspoon pepper

Melt margarine in a 1½-quart pot; add onions and green pepper and stir over medium heat 5 minutes. Add remaining ingredients; mix well and stir over medium heat for 5 more minutes.

Nutritive values per serving: CHO 16 gm., PRO 3 gm., FAT 4 gm., Calories 96, Sodium 491 mg.

Food Exchanges per serving: 1 Bread Exchange plus 1 Fat Exchange.

Low-sodium diets: Omit salt. Use unsalted margarine, unsalted canned corn, and unsalted canned tomatoes.

Green Beans Almondine

4 servings (yield: 2 cups)   1 serving: ½ cup

1 package (9 ounces) French-cut green beans
⅓ cup boiling water
½ teaspoon salt
1½ tablespoons margarine
1 tablespoon slivered almonds

Cook green beans in salted boiling water in a small covered saucepan, separating beans with a fork, 8 minutes until crisp-tender. Meanwhile heat margarine in a small pan; sauté almonds in margarine until they are golden and margarine is slightly browned. Drain beans and toss with almond mixture.

Nutritive values per serving: CHO 4 gm., PRO 2 gm., FAT 5 gm., Calories 65, Sodium 187 mg.

Food Exchanges per serving: 1 Vegetable Exchange plus 1 Fat Exchange.

Low-sodium diets: Omit salt. Use unsalted margarine.

Green Beans Italiano

5 servings (yield: 4 cups)   1 serving: ¾ cup

1 tablespoon margarine
1 medium cooking onion
2 cloves garlic, crushed
1 small can (8 ounces) tomatoes
1 can (16 ounces) cut green beans
¼ cup chopped sweet green pepper
¼ teaspoon salt
½ teaspoon crushed oregano
1 tablespoon wine vinegar

Melt margarine in a heavy, deep saucepan. Peel onion and slice crosswise in thin rings; sauté onions and garlic in melted margarine. Stir over medium heat with a wooden spoon until onions are tender but not browned. Cut tomatoes into bite-sized pieces. Add to onions with tomato liquid, green beans and their liquid, and all remaining ingredients. Mix well. Bring to a boil and simmer gently about 10 minutes to blend flavors.

Nutritive values per serving: CHO 9 gm., PRO 2 gm., FAT 3 gm., Calories 60, Sodium 411 mg.

Food Exchanges per serving: 2 Vegetable Exchanges plus ½ Fat Exchange.

Low-sodium diets: Omit salt. Use unsalted margarine, low-sodium canned tomatoes, and low-sodium canned green beans.

Mary's Easy Mushrooms

7 servings (yield: 3½ cups)   1 serving: ½ cup

1 pound fresh mushrooms
1 tablespoon margarine, broken in bits
¼ teaspoon salt
Dash pepper

Preheat oven to 350° F. (180° C.). Wash mushrooms thoroughly and remove tough tips from bottom of stem. Cut a large piece of aluminum foil; place mushrooms in the middle of the foil, dot with margarine, and sprinkle with salt and pepper. Fold foil around mushrooms; seal package tightly by crimping edges. Bake for 20 to 30 minutes in oven or on a barbecue grill. Open package very carefully to avoid spilling the delicious juices from the mushrooms. These mushrooms with their juices are great with steak or roast beef.

Nutritive values per serving: CHO 3 gm., PRO 2 gm., FAT 1 gm., Calories 33, Sodium 92 mg.

Food Exchange per serving: 1 Vegetable Exchange.

Low-sodium diets: Omit salt. Use unsalted margarine.

Yummy Onions

5 servings (yield: 2½ cups)   1 serving: ½ cup

4 cups onions, cut in wedges
1 cup water
1 chicken bouillon cube
¼ cup finely diced sweet green pepper
1 tablespoon vegetable oil
½ teaspoon salt
½ teaspoon Italian seasoning
¼ teaspoon garlic powder
Dash of ground cloves

Combine all ingredients in a saucepan. Cover tightly and simmer over medium heat 25 minutes.

Nutritive values per serving: CHO 8 gm., PRO 2 gm., FAT 3 gm., Calories 62, Sodium 416 mg.

Food Exchanges per serving: 1½ Vegetable Exchanges plus ½ Fat Exchange.

Low-sodium diets: Omit salt. Use low-sodium chicken bouillon cube.

Sautéed Sweet Peppers

This very colorful vegetable may be served alone but it's beautiful over a beef patty or over a plain omelet.

6 servings (yield: 3 cups) 1 serving: ½ cup

2 medium (9 ounces) sweet green peppers
2 medium (9 ounces) sweet red peppers
2 tablespoons margarine
2 tablespoons water
½ teaspoon salt
½ teaspoon dried basil or 1 tablespoon fresh chopped basil
⅛ teaspoon coarsely ground pepper

Wash peppers; remove stems, seeds, and cores. Cut peppers into 1-inch squares. Heat margarine in a large frying pan over medium heat; add peppers and cook 3 to 4 minutes, stirring often. Add water and continue stirring and cooking another 4 to 5 minutes until peppers are crisp-tender. Add seasonings and serve.

Nutritive values per serving: CHO 3 gm., PRO 1 gm., FAT 4 gm., Calories 47, Sodium 235 mg.

Food Exchanges per serving: 1 Vegetable Exchange plus ½ Fat Exchange.

Low-sodium diets: Omit salt. Use unsalted margarine.

Ratatouille

This versatile vegetable mixture is great served either hot or cold. Mary likes to serve it warm on toast points as an appetizer or chilled on Boston lettuce with additional capers on top. She always makes enough so that she can serve it hot once and cold once.

16 servings (yield: 8 cups)   1 serving: ½ cup

¼ cup olive oil
4 tablespoons margarine
3 cloves garlic, crushed
3 medium onions, coarsely chopped (2 cups)
1 medium (1 pound) eggplant, peeled and cubed
2 medium sweet green peppers, cored and sliced (8 to 9 ounces)
2 medium zucchini, sliced (about 12 ounces)
3 tablespoons flour
1 can (16 ounces) tomatoes, cut up with liquid
¾ cup water
1 can (6 ounces) tomato paste
1 teaspoon sugar
1 teaspoon salt
½ teaspoon coarsely ground pepper
¼ cup chopped parsley
2 teaspoons capers, drained

Heat the oil and margarine in a large pot. Add garlic and onions and cook until onions are translucent. Add eggplant, green pepper, and zucchini, and cook, stirring often, until vegetables wilt. Sprinkle flour over vegetable mixture; stir in tomatoes with liquid, water, and tomato paste. Cover and cook over low heat 20 minutes, stirring often to prevent sticking to the bottom of pot. Add remaining ingredients and cook uncovered 10 more minutes; stir often.

Nutritive values per serving: CHO 9 gm., PRO 2 gm., FAT 6 gm.,
                                 Calories 97, Sodium 282 mg.
Food Exchanges per serving: 2 Vegetable Exchanges plus 1 Fat
                                 Exchange.

Low-sodium diets: Omit salt and capers. Use unsalted marga-
                                 rine, 4 small fresh tomatoes for the canned
                                 tomatoes, and unsalted tomato paste.

Baked Spinach Casserole

5 servings (yield: 2½ cups) 1 serving: ½ cup

2 packages (10 ounces each) frozen chopped spinach
2 eggs, beaten
1 tablespoon flour
½ teaspoon salt
⅛ teaspoon pepper
⅛ teaspoon garlic powder
2 teaspoons lemon juice
½ teaspoon vegetable oil (to oil casserole)

Preheat oven to 350° F. (180° C.). Cook spinach as directed on package except simmer only 3 minutes; drain. To beaten eggs add flour, seasonings, and lemon juice; beat with a hand beater. Add cooked spinach and mix well. Turn into lightly oiled 1-quart casserole. Bake uncovered for 20 to 25 minutes.

Nutritive values per serving: CHO 5 gm., PRO 6 gm., FAT 4 gm., Calories 74, Sodium 291 mg.

Food Exchanges per serving: 1 Vegetable Exchange plus ½ High-Fat Meat Exchange.

Low-sodium diets: Omit salt.

Spinach with Nutmeg

5 servings (yield: 2½ cups)   1 serving: ½ cup

2 packages (10 ounces) frozen chopped spinach
1 cup boiling water
½ teaspoon salt
½ cup Lemon Mayonnaise (see Index)
¼ teaspoon coarsely ground pepper
¼ teaspoon ground nutmeg

Cook spinach in salted boiling water in a saucepan. Separate spinach with a fork; cook over moderate heat, covered, 8 to 10 minutes or until tender. Drain in a strainer, pressing out excess liquid with the back of a wooden spoon. Return spinach to pan; stir in Lemon Mayonnaise, pepper, and nutmeg. Reheat gently 2 minutes.

Nutritive values per serving: CHO 4 gm., PRO 3 gm., FAT 1 gm., Calories 34, Sodium 479 mg.

Food Exchange per serving: 1 Vegetable Exchange.

Low-sodium diets: Omit salt in recipe and in preparing Lemon Mayonnaise.

Mashed Winter Squash

Use butternut, Hubbard, or acorn squash as you prefer.

4 servings (yield: 2 cups)   1 serving: ½ cup

1¾ pounds winter squash
½ teaspoon vegetable oil
1½ tablespoons margarine, cut in pieces
Cinnamon for garnish (optional)

Preheat oven to 350° F. (180° C.). Cut each squash in quarters lengthwise; scoop out seeds and discard. Score yellow meaty part of each quarter with a knife. Brush bottom of a shallow baking pan with the vegetable oil. Place squash pieces in pan with skin sides up. Bake 45 minutes or until very tender. Carefully remove skin from squash and put squash pulp into a bowl; beat until fluffy; add margarine and beat it in well. If desired, garnish with sprinkle of cinnamon.

Nutritive values per serving: CHO 14 gm., PRO 2 gm., FAT 4 gm., Calories 95, Sodium 72 mg.

Food Exchanges per serving: 1 Bread Exchange plus 1 Fat Exchange.

Low-sodium diets: Use unsalted margarine.

Pineapple Squash

4 servings   1 serving: ½ stuffed squash

2 small (2 pounds) acorn squash, 3½ inch diameter
1 can (8 ounces) unsweetened crushed pineapple, with juice
2 teaspoons margarine
½ teaspoon cinnamon
Hot water

Preheat oven to 375° F. (190° C.). Cut each squash in half; scoop out and discard seeds and pulp. Trim tip off bottom if necessary so that each squash cup stands up straight. Fill each squash cup with ¼ cup crushed pineapple, ½ teaspoon margarine, and a sprinkle of cinnamon. Put squash into a flat baking dish and pour hot water around bottoms of squash to a depth of ½ inch. Cover pan tightly with foil. Bake 1 hour or until squash is tender and can be easily pierced with a fork.

Nutritive values per serving: CHO 28 gm., PRO 3 gm., FAT 2 gm., Calories 129, Sodium 26 mg.

Food Exchanges per serving: 1 Bread Exchange plus 1 Fruit Exchange plus ½ Fat Exchange.

Low-sodium diets: This recipe is excellent.

Baked Tomatoes

4 servings   1 serving: 1 tomato

4 small (about 1 pound) tomatoes
1 slice bread, finely crumbled (¾ cup soft crumbs)
½ teaspoon herb or Italian seasoning
½ teaspoon salt
⅛ teaspoon coarsely ground black pepper
1 tablespoon finely cut green onion
1 teaspoon margarine, melted

Preheat oven to 350° F. (180° C.). Wash tomatoes and cut a thin slice off top; scoop out pulp into a bowl, leaving good "shells." Mix pulp, ½ cup of the bread crumbs, seasonings, and green onion. Place tomato "shells" in an 8-inch-square pan or a pie pan. Divide pulp mixture evenly between the tomatoes, placing in hollows carefully. Mix melted margarine with remaining ¼ cup bread crumbs and sprinkle on top of tomatoes. Bake about 25 minutes, until tomatoes are tender.

Nutritive values per serving: CHO 8 gm., PRO 2 gm., FAT 1 gm., Calories 48, Sodium 316 mg.

Food Exchange per serving: 1 Vegetable Exchange *or* 1 Fruit Exchange.

Low-sodium diets: Omit salt.

Mashed Turnips

4 servings (yield: 2 cups)   1 serving: ½ cup

1 pound turnips, without tops
2 cups boiling water
1½ tablespoons margarine
½ teaspoon salt
⅛ teaspoon black pepper
Paprika or chopped parsley for garnish

Remove tops and root ends, and pare turnips; cut turnips in small cubes. Measure boiling water into a small, heavy saucepan. Add cubed turnips; cover pan, bring to a boil, turn heat low, and cook for about 20 minutes or until tender. Drain any remaining water, but most of it should be cooked away. Mash turnips thoroughly with a hand masher or an electric beater; add margarine, salt, and pepper. Beat until blended and fluffy. If garnish is desired, sprinkle paprika or finely cut parsley on top.

Nutritive values per serving: CHO 6 gm., PRO 1 gm., FAT 5 gm., Calories 64, Sodium 225 mg.

Food Exchanges per serving: 1 Vegetable Exchange plus 1 Fat Exchange.

Low-sodium diets: Omit salt. Use unsalted margarine.

Vegetable Medley

5 servings (yield: 3⅓ cups)   1 serving: ⅔ cup

1 can (8¼ ounces) julienne carrots
1 can (8¾ ounces) French-cut green beans
1 tablespoon vegetable oil
1 cup thinly sliced cauliflowerets
½ cup sliced onion rings
Water
2 teaspoons cornstarch
2 chicken bouillon cubes
2 tablespoons cheese cracker crumbs

Drain carrots and green beans, saving liquids. Heat vegetable oil in a 10- or 12-inch frying pan; add cauliflower and onion rings and stir-fry over medium heat for 3 minutes. To the drained liquids from the canned vegetables add enough water to make a total of 1 cup of liquid. Add about ¼ cup of this to cornstarch and mix until smooth. Add remaining liquid, mix well, then add with the canned vegetables to mixture in frying pan; mix well. Add chicken bouillon cubes. Cook and stir over medium heat until bouillon cubes are dissolved and sauce is thickened. Cover pan and let "steam" over low heat for another 2 minutes. To serve, turn into serving dish and scatter cheese cracker crumbs on top.

Nutritive values per serving: CHO 9 gm., PRO 2 gm., FAT 3 gm., Calories 70, Sodium 598 mg.

Food Exchanges per serving: 2 Vegetable Exchanges plus ½ Fat Exchange.

Low-sodium diets: Use low-sodium bouillon cubes and unsalted canned vegetables.

Zucchini Sauté

4 servings (yield: 2⅔ cups)   1 serving: ⅔ cup

2 to 3 medium (1 pound) zucchini
1 tablespoon vegetable oil
½ cup thinly sliced red onion
¼ teaspoon oregano or basil
¼ teaspoon salt
Dash of black pepper

Clean and slice zucchini into thin strips or bite-sized pieces. Heat oil in a large frying pan. Add onions and stir-fry quickly until onions are translucent, not browned. Add zucchini, cover frying pan, and cook 3 to 4 minutes, until zucchini is wilted. Sprinkle with all seasonings and mix well.

Nutritive values per serving: CHO 5 gm., PRO 1 gm., FAT 4 gm., Calories 52, Sodium 136 mg.

Food Exchanges per serving: 1 Vegetable Exchange plus ½ Fat Exchange.

Low-sodium diets: Omit salt.

Zucchini and Tomatoes au Gratin

10 servings (yield: 5 cups)   1 serving: ½ cup

1½ pounds zucchini
1 can (10 ounces) tomatoes with liquid
1 tablespoon vegetable oil
¾ cup thinly sliced onion rings
½ cup tomato juice
¼ teaspoon salt
⅛ teaspoon pepper
½ cup grated Parmesan cheese

Preheat oven to 350° F. (180° C.). Cut zucchini crosswise in thin slices. Cut tomatoes in bite-sized pieces. Use ½ teaspoon of oil to prepare casserole. Heat remaining oil in a large frying pan. Add onion rings and cook over medium heat, stirring until limp. Add zucchini slices, cover, and cook over low heat 5 minutes. Add tomatoes, juice from can, tomato juice, salt, and pepper; mix carefully. Turn into a lightly oiled 1½- to 2-quart casserole. Sprinkle with grated cheese. Bake about 20 minutes until top is golden brown.

Nutritive values per serving: CHO 5 gm., PRO 3 gm., FAT 3 gm., Calories 58, Sodium 119 mg.

Food Exchanges per serving: 1 Vegetable Exchange plus ½ Fat Exchange.

Low-sodium diets: Omit salt. Use unsalted canned tomatoes and unsalted tomato juice.

34

Desserts

Sherry Ambrosia

6 servings (yield: 3 cups)   1 serving: ½ cup

⅔ cup (110 grams) fresh orange sections
1 cup (200 grams) fresh grapefruit sections
1 cup (125 grams) diced red apples
2 tablespoons dry sherry
1 teaspoon lemon juice
Artificial sweetener to substitute for 2 teaspoons sugar (optional)
⅓ cup (50 grams) sliced bananas
2 tablespoons shredded coconut
3 maraschino cherries, drained

Cut orange sections in halves, grapefruit sections in quarters, and cored (but not pared) red-skin apples in small, bite-sized cubes. Measure and weigh fruits, then mix well with sherry and lemon juice. If desired, add a few drops of liquid artificial sweetener. Turn into a jar, cover, and chill for 1 hour or longer. Just before serving, add bananas; mix well. Spoon into 6 individual dessert dishes. With scissors, cut coconut into small pieces; scatter on top of fruits. Slice maraschino cherries; place a few slices on top of coconut.

Nutritive values per serving: CHO 12 gm., PRO 1 gm., FAT 1 gm., Calories 59, Sodium 1 mg.

Food Exchanges per serving: 1½ Fruit Exchanges.

Low-sodium diets: This recipe is excellent.

Granny Smith Applesauce

This recipe was kitchen tested in June, early in the new apple season, with Granny Smith apples, which were very firm, large, and yielded 3 cups sauce for 4 apples. The sauce was a "solid" pack.

9 servings (yield: 3 cups)   1 serving: ⅓ cup

2 pounds firm Granny Smith apples
2 tablespoons lemon juice
1 cup water
¼ teaspoon cinnamon
Artificial sweetener to substitute for 9 teaspoons sugar

Pare apples very thin, preferably with a vegetable parer. Remove cores; cut apples into 8 to 12 slices, then in bite-sized pieces. Measure 6 cups (660 grams) into a large, heavy pot; add lemon juice and water; mix well. Bring to a boil; cover and cook gently until apples are very soft and tender. Remove from heat; add cinnamon and artificial sweetener; mix thoroughly with a wooden spoon (a metal spoon may darken the sauce). Pack into jars, cover, and store in refrigerator. Serve warm or chilled.

Nutritive values per serving: CHO 10 gm., PRO 0, FAT 0, Calories 40, Sodium 6 mg.

Food Exchange per serving: 1 Fruit Exchange.

Low-sodium diets: This recipe is excellent.

Pink Applesauce

4 servings (yield: 2 cups)   1 serving: ½ cup

1 pound red skin apples (Jonathan or McIntosh)
1½ cups water
1 tablespoon lemon juice
⅛ teaspoon cinnamon
¹⁄₁₆ teaspoon mace
Artificial sweetener to substitute for 2 to 3 tablespoons sugar

Wash apples, cut in quarters; leave skin on, but remove and discard cores. Cut apples into small cubes; there will be about 3 cups (330 grams). Place apples in pot; add water and lemon juice. Cover, bring to a boil. Cook gently over medium heat, stirring occasionally, until apples are soft (about 8 to 10 minutes). Remove from heat; add cinnamon, mace, and sweetener; mix well. Turn into a pint jar; cool, cover, and store in refrigerator.

Nutritive values per serving: CHO 12 gm., PRO 0, FAT 0, Calories 49, Sodium 1 mg.

Food Exchange per serving: 1 Fruit Exchange.

Low-sodium diets: This recipe is excellent.

Grand Marnier Fruit Cup

4 servings (yield: 2 cups)   1 serving: ½ cup

1 small fresh peach or nectarine
2 small purple plums
1 small red apple
24 green Thompson seedless grapes
2 teaspoons lemon juice
Artificial sweetener to substitute for 2 tablespoons sugar
1½ tablespoons Grand Marnier

Wash fruit. Peel peach. Remove stones from peach or nectarine and plums and core from apple. Cut grapes in half; cut remaining fruit in small bite-sized pieces. Mix fruits well with remaining ingredients. Turn into a jar, cover, and chill for a few hours to blend flavors.

Nutritive values per serving: CHO 12 gm., PRO 0, FAT 0, Calories 58, Sodium 1 mg.

Food Exchanges per serving: 1 Fruit Exchange plus ½ Fat Exchange (to account for calories from the alcohol in the Grand Marnier).

Low-sodium diets: This recipe is excellent.

Poached Pears Delight

5 servings (yield: 10 halves plus   1 serving: 2 pear halves plus
  1 cup liquid)   3 to 4 tablespoons liquid

5 (1 pound) prepared small, just underripe pears (D'Anjou, Bartlett, or Bosc)
3½ cups water
2 tablespoons lemon juice
2 teaspoons imitation rum flavor
1 teaspoon pure vanilla extract
1¼ teaspoons pure orange flavor
Artificial sweetener to substitute for 2½ tablespoons sugar

Pare, halve lengthwise, and core the pears; the total weight of the 10 halves will be approximately 330 grams (11 ounces). Put prepared pear halves, water, and lemon juice in a saucepan. Bring to a boil, turn heat down, and let simmer gently 20 to 22 minutes or until pears are tender but firm. Remove from heat. Lift pears out carefully with a spoon and place in a pint jar or bowl. Add all flavorings and artificial sweetener to hot liquid; stir to blend well. Pour on top of pears. Cover tightly. Chill and store in refrigerator.

Nutritive values per serving: CHO 10 gm., PRO 0, FAT 0, Calories 41, Sodium 1 mg.

Food Exchange per serving: 1 Fruit Exchange when served plain. If served with Vanilla Crème Fraîche (*see* Index) or with ladyfingers, count their values in addition.

Low-sodium diets: This recipe is excellent.

Stewed Rhubarb

Frozen, unsweetened rhubarb is sold in 1-pound packages. The amount of fresh rhubarb to pick or buy, in order to end up with the same quantity—4 cups uncooked—depends upon how much top and bottom is left on before cleaning and cutting. Be sure all leaves are removed because they are poisonous.

4 servings (yield: 2 cups)   1 serving: ½ cup

1 pound (4 cups) diced fresh or frozen rhubarb
¼ cup water
Artificial sweetener to substitute for 18 teaspoons of sugar*

Place diced rhubarb and water in a deep saucepan. Cover and bring to a boil; turn heat down and simmer gently until rhubarb is very tender, about 10 minutes, stirring occasionally. Remove from heat, add artificial sweetener and mix well. Turn into a pint jar. Cover and store in refrigerator.

Nutritive values per serving: CHO 4 gm., PRO 0.5 gm., FAT 0, Calories 16, Sodium 2 mg.

Food Exchange per serving: ½ Fruit Exchange.

Low-sodium diets: This recipe is excellent.

   * The amount of artificial sweetener required is largely dependent upon the acidity or "sour" taste of the rhubarb you use. Taste and adjust amount of sweetener accordingly.

Peter's Favorite Strawberries

Mary's husband Peter particularly likes this simple but elegant dessert. Mary serves it in champagne or brandy glasses.

4 servings (yield: 3 cups)   1 serving: ¾ cup

1 pint ripe, very red strawberries
1 medium (200 grams) orange
2 tablespoons orange juice
2 tablespoons sweet vermouth
Artificial sweetener to substitute for 3 teaspoons sugar (optional)

Wash and hull strawberries; cut each in half. Slice ends off orange; quarter orange lengthwise and slice orange wedges crosswise with rinds left on, as thin as possible. Put strawberries and oranges in a bowl; mix well. Mix together the orange juice and sweet vermouth and drizzle over fruit mixture; stir to mix. Check to see if berries have enough natural sweetness for your taste; if not, add artificial sweetener. Cover bowl and chill in refrigerator 2 hours before serving; stir gently several times to blend flavors.

Nutritive values per serving: CHO 13 gm., PRO 1 gm., FAT 0, Calories 62, Sodium 1 mg.

Food Exchanges per serving: 1½ Fruit Exchanges. If you are only allowed 1 Fruit Exchange, serve only ½ cup of this recipe.

Low-sodium diets: This recipe is excellent.

Rich Strawberry Trifle

6 servings (yield: 3 cups)   1 serving: ½ cup plus 4 vanilla wafers

1¼ cups Phony Whipped Cream (*see* Index)
1 pint (300 grams) fresh strawberries
Artificial sweetener to substitute for 1 tablespoon sugar
2 tablespoons Grand Marnier
1½ cups whole milk
4 medium eggs
⅛ teaspoon salt
1¼ teaspoons vanilla
¼ teaspoon pure orange flavoring
Artificial sweetener to substitute for ¼ cup sugar
24 (100 grams) vanilla wafers

Prepare Phony Whipped Cream. Chill it. Meanwhile, wash strawberries, reserving 6 whole berries with hulls for garnish. Slice and
quarter remaining berries and mix with artificial sweetener to
substitute for 1 tablespoon sugar; add Grand Marnier; mix well,
cover, set aside. Scald milk in the top of a double boiler. Beat eggs
and salt slightly. Pour hot milk on top of egg mixture very slowly,
stirring constantly. Return mixture to the top of the double boiler.
Place over simmering water (water should not touch bottom of top
part). Cook, stirring constantly, until mixture coats a metal spoon.
Immediately remove from over simmering water; add vanilla,
orange flavoring, and artificial sweetener to substitute for ¼ cup
sugar. Cool custard well; fold in 1 cup of Phony Whipped Cream;
blend carefully. Arrange 16 vanilla wafers on bottom and around
sides of a large glass dessert bowl (or 3 in each of six individual
dessert servers). Spread half of the strawberries on top, then half of
the custard mixture. Repeat with remaining vanilla wafers, then
strawberries, and finally custard. Cover with clear plastic. Chill for
several hours. When ready to serve, garnish with spoonfuls of
remaining Phony Whipped Cream and reserved whole strawberries.

Nutritive values per serving: CHO 22 gm., PRO 8 gm., FAT 10
                                  gm., Calories 223, Sodium 166 mg.

Food Exchanges per serving: 1 Milk Exchange plus 1 Fruit Ex-
                                  change plus 2 Fat Exchanges.

Low-sodium diets: Omit salt.

Graham Cracker Pie Shell

Do not use packaged graham cracker crumbs for this recipe because their carbohydrate content is higher than that of graham wafers.

8 servings (yield: 9-inch pie shell)   1 serving: ⅛ pie shell

7 (100 grams) large, plain graham wafers (each 2½ by 5 inches across)
3 tablespoons margarine, melted

Break graham wafers in small pieces, place in a plastic bag, fasten opening with a bag tie, and press with a rolling pin or a large jar to make crumbs. Continue until all crumbs are fine (total of 1¼ cups). Empty into a bowl. Melt the margarine, add to crumbs, and mix well with a fork. Set aside 2 tablespoons to use later as the garnish on the pie filling. Using the back of a spoon, press remainder of crumb mixture evenly on bottom and sides of a 9-inch pie plate. Chill in refrigerator for 3 hours or longer before filling.

Nutritive values:
   entire pie shell—   CHO 73 gm., PRO 8 gm., FAT 44 gm., Calories 691, Sodium 1085 mg.

   per serving (crust only)—   CHO 9 gm., PRO 1 gm., FAT 5 gm., Calories 86, Sodium 136 mg.

Food Exchanges per serving
   (crust only):   ½ Bread Exchange plus 1 Fat Exchange.

Low-sodium diets: Use unsalted margarine.

Vanilla Wafer Crumb Crust

Use this unbaked shell for Chocolate Pie, Jo's Cranberry Pie (see Index), or for other fillings.

8 servings (yield: 9-inch pie shell)   1 serving: ⅛ pie shell

2 tablespoons margarine, melted
30 vanilla wafers (1¾ inch diameter)
¼ teaspoon pure vanilla flavor

Prepare a 9-inch pie plate by rubbing inside, bottom, and sides with ½ teaspoon of the margarine; set aside. Crush vanilla wafers to make very fine crumbs (1¼ cups). Place crumbs in a large bowl; combine vanilla and melted margarine and drizzle all over crumbs. Mix thoroughly with a blending fork to make sure all is well blended. Remove about 2 tablespoons of crumb mixture and set aside to use if desired as a garnish on top of pie. With back of a large spoon, press remaining crumbs evenly all over bottom and sides of prepared pie pan. Chill in refrigerator 2 hours or longer before filling.

Nutritive values:
    entire pie shell—   CHO 90 gm., PRO 7 gm., FAT 31 gm., Calories 657, Sodium 443 mg.

    per serving (crust
    only)—   CHO 11 gm., PRO 1 gm., FAT 4 gm., Calories 82, Sodium 55 mg.

Food Exchanges per serving
    (crust only):   1 Fruit Exchange plus 1 Fat Exchange.

Low-sodium diets: Use unsalted margarine.

Banana Cream Pie

8 servings (yield: 9-inch pie)   1 serving: ⅛ pie

1 Vanilla Wafer Crumb Crust (*see* Index)
1½ teaspoons granulated gelatin
¼ cup cold water
1½ cups hot skim milk
¼ cup flour
¼ teaspoon salt
½ cup cold skim milk
2 eggs, beaten
Artificial sweetener to substitute for 9 teaspoons sugar
1½ teaspoons pure vanilla
1 pound firm-ripe bananas

Prepare piecrust first because it should be chilled 2 hours or longer before filling. Soak gelatin in cold water and set aside. Heat 1½ cups milk in the top of a double boiler over simmering water. In a small bowl combine flour, salt, and ½ cup cold milk; mix until smooth and without lumps Slowly pour ½ cup of the hot milk into the bowl with the flour mixture; stir to mix well. Then slowly pour contents of the bowl back into the pot of hot milk. Cook and stir over simmering water until thick and smooth. Pour mixture slowly on top of beaten eggs, stirring constantly. Return to top of double boiler. Cook and stir over simmering water about 4 minutes; remove from heat. Add gelatin, artificial sweetener, and vanilla; mix well to dissolve gelatin. Cool and chill until mixture begins to gel. Peel bananas, slice thin and measure 1½ cups (225 grams). Arrange 1 cup sliced bananas in bottom of pie shell, then very carefully spoon and pour filling on top evenly. Arrange remaining ½ cup sliced bananas on top and garnish with the vanilla crumbs saved when making pie shell. Cover whole pie carefully with plastic wrap. Chill 2 to 3 hours until set and firm. For serving, cut in eight equal pieces.

Nutritive values per serving: CHO 24 gm., PRO 6 gm., FAT 5 gm., Calories 162, Sodium 168 mg.

Food Exchanges per serving: 1 Milk Exchange plus 1 Fruit Exchange plus 1 Fat Exchange.

Low-sodium diets: Omit salt. Use unsalted margarine in piecrust recipe.

Chocolate Pie

Mary's seven-year-old Rachel, a most particular young lady, approves of this one, probably because it is chocolate and is a pie!

6 servings (yield: 9-inch pie)   1 serving: ⅙ pie

1 Vanilla Wafer Crumb Crust (*see* Index)
1¼ cups firmly packed Chocolate Pudding Mix (*see* Index)
2¼ cups cold water
¾ teaspoon pure vanilla
Artificial sweetener to substitute for 10 teaspoons sugar

Prepare Vanilla Wafer Crumb Crust (reserve 2 tablespoons crumb mixture), pack into a 9-inch pie shell, and chill in refrigerator at least 2 hours before making filling. Measure dry pudding mix into a heavy saucepan; add water slowly, mixing well. Stir constantly over moderate heat until bubbling boil is reached around outside edge. Remove from heat; stir in vanilla and artificial sweetener to blend well. Let cool for 10 minutes, stirring three or four times. Spoon slowly and carefully into chilled pie shell; smooth with a small spatula. Scatter the 2 tablespoons crumb mixture on top as garnish. Cover pie carefully but completely with plastic wrap. Chill in refrigerator at least 2 hours before serving. If desired, garnish with Phony Whipped Cream (*see* Index).

Nutritive values per serving: CHO 27 gm., PRO 4 gm., FAT 6 gm., Calories 171, Sodium 111 mg.

Food Exchanges per serving: 2 Bread Exchanges plus 1 Fat Exchange.

Low-sodium diets·   This recipe is fine unless sodium is severely restricted, but use unsalted margarine in piecrust recipe.

Jo's Cranberry Pie

This is a really great pie and is shown on the cover of this book. Josephine Anderson's original recipe is the Thanksgiving favorite at Mary's home and is not for diabetics. But Kay has made a very good "diabetic copy." Calculations include the topping as well as the crust!

8 servings (yield: 9-inch pie)   1 serving: ⅛ pie

1 Vanilla Wafer Crumb Crust (*see* Index)
1 tablespoon granulated gelatin
2 cups cold water
3 cups raw fresh or frozen cranberries
¼ teaspoon grated orange rind
¼ teaspoon pure orange flavor
Artificial sweetener to substitute for 27 teaspoons of sugar
1½ cups Phony Whipped Cream (*see* Index)

Make crumb crust according to recipe and chill in refrigerator at least 2 hours before filling. Soak gelatin in ½ cup cold water; set aside. Pick over fresh or frozen cranberries, wash, and measure; put in a deep, heavy saucepan with 1½ cups water and orange rind. Cook over moderate heat until all cranberries pop, stirring occasionally. Remove from heat. Stir in gelatin, orange flavor, and artificial sweetener; mix until gelatin is dissolved. Let cool for about 30 minutes, stirring occasionally. Taste to see if enough sweetener has been added because cranberries vary greatly in tartness. Spoon carefully and slowly into piecrust and smooth evenly with the back of a spoon. Chill in refrigerator while you make the Phony Whipped Cream. After Cream is made and chilled in freezer for 15 minutes, measure 1½ cups and spread on top of pie, smoothing and swirling evenly. Chill in refrigerator for 3 to 4 hours before serving.

Nutritive values per serving: CHO 16 gm., PRO 3 gm., FAT 6 gm., Calories 125, Sodium 68 mg.

Food Exchanges per serving: 1 Bread Exchange plus 1 Fat Exchange.

Low-sodium diets: Use unsalted margarine in piecrust recipe.

Lemon Cheese Pie

Some of Kay's nondiabetic friends asked for double-sized servings of this one!

8 servings (yield: 9-inch pie)   1 serving: ⅛ pie

1 Graham Cracker Pie Shell (*see* Index)
1½ tablespoons granulated gelatin
½ cup cold water
1 cup skim milk
3 medium eggs, beaten
¼ teaspoon salt
1 tablespoon grated lemon rind
⅓ cup lemon juice
½ teaspoon pure lemon extract
Artificial sweetener to substitute for ½ cup sugar
1 pound (2 cups) small curd cream-style cottage cheese
3 to 4 fresh strawberries or thin lemon slices for garnish

Soak gelatin in cold water. Scald milk in top of a double boiler. Pour slowly on top of gently beaten eggs and salt, stirring constantly. Return to top of the double boiler; cook over slowly simmering water, stirring constantly, until mixture coats spoon. Remove from heat. Turn into a bowl; add gelatin, lemon rind, lemon juice, lemon extract, and artificial sweetener; mix well until gelatin is dissolved. Chill until mixture is the consistency of unbeaten egg whites; stir gently several times while chilling. Add cottage cheese. Beat with an electric mixer at high speed for 8 to 10 minutes. If filling thins, chill for 5 to 10 minutes. Turn into prepared 9-inch Graham Cracker Pie Shell. Sprinkle reserved 2 tablespoons cracker crumbs on top; garnish with sliced strawberries or lemons. Chill 3 hours or longer.

Nutritive values per serving: CHO 13 gm., PRO 11 gm., FAT 9 gm., Calories 177, Sodium 444 mg.

Food Exchanges per serving: 1 Bread Exchange plus 1½ Medium-Fat Meat Exchanges.

Low-sodium diets: Omit salt. Use unsalted cottage cheese if available. Use unsalted margarine in the piecrust recipe.

Holiday Pumpkin Chiffon Pie

8 servings (yield: 9-inch pie)   1 serving: ⅛ pie

1 Graham Cracker Pie Shell (*see* Index)
1 tablespoon granulated gelatin
½ cup cold water
3 eggs, separated
½ cup whole milk
1¼ cups (306 grams) solid pack canned pumpkin
½ teaspoon salt
¼ teaspoon nutmeg
¾ teaspoon cinnamon
½ teaspoon ginger
½ teaspoon allspice
Artificial sweetener to substitute for ½ cup sugar
2 tablespoons sugar
2 teaspoons brandy

Dissolve gelatin in cold water; set aside. Beat egg yolks lightly, stir in milk, pumpkin, salt, and spices; blend well. Cook in the top of a double boiler, stirring constantly until thick and smooth, about 8 minutes. Remove from heat, add gelatin and artificial sweetener, stir until completely dissolved. Cool, then chill in refrigerator until mixture thickens to consistency of unbeaten egg white. Remove from refrigerator. Beat egg whites until soft peaks form. Add sugar and brandy gradually to egg whites, beating constantly until stiff, glossy, and shiny. Fold carefully but thoroughly into pumpkin mixture. Turn carefully into the prepared pie shell; scatter reserved 2 tablespoons graham cracker crumbs on top as garnish. Chill about 8 hours. Slice in 8 equal portions.

Nutritive values per serving: CHO 16 gm., PRO 5 gm., FAT 8 gm., Calories 153, Sodium 387 mg.

Food Exchanges per serving: 1½ Fruit Exchanges plus 1 High-Fat Meat Exchange.

Low-sodium diets: Omit salt. Use unsalted margarine in piecrust recipe. When available, use unsalted canned pumpkin for filling.

Apple Cobbler

8 servings (yield: 9-inch pie)   1 serving: ⅛ pie

1¾ pounds (about 4) medium-sized cooking apples
  (Jonathans or Wealthies)
1½ tablespoons lemon juice
½ teaspoon grated lemon rind
1 tablespoon cornstarch
1 teaspoon apple pie spice
¼ teaspoon salt
Artificial sweetener to substitute for 12 teaspoons sugar
½ cup flour
3 tablespoons margarine or butter

Preheat oven to 425° F. (218° C.). Prepare inside of a 9-inch pie plate with vegetable pan coating (spray or solid). Pare apples, remove cores, and cut apples in ⅛-inch slices; measure 4 cups (600 grams). Combine apple slices, lemon juice, and rind. Combine cornstarch, spice, ⅛ teaspoon salt, and artificial sweetener; mix thoroughly. Add to apples and stir lightly with a fork to coat all slices. Spread apples evenly in prepared pie plate; set aside. Mix together flour and remaining ⅛ teaspoon salt. Cut in margarine or butter with pastry blender or fork until crumbly; scatter all over top of apples. Bake about 35 minutes or until top is golden brown. Serve warm.

Nutritive values per serving: CHO 16 gm., PRO 1 gm., FAT 5 gm., Calories 106, Sodium 87 mg.

Food Exchanges per serving: 1 Bread Exchange plus 1 Fat Exchange.

Low-sodium diets: Omit salt. Use unsalted margarine or butter.

Fruit-Flavored Gels

Because sugar-free gelatin desserts are so tasty and popular on menus for diabetics, the following recipes are included. These will be especially useful if you are unable to get commercial fruit-flavored gelatin products prepared for special diets. Because of the wide differences in the carbohydrate values of the different fruit juices, it is necessary to have separate recipes for each fruit gel. The same is true for the amount of artificial sweetener you use to substitute for the sugar.

Here are a few simple rules to guide you in making fruit-flavored gelatin desserts. Our recipes are tested and are successful as well as delicious, but if you want to try other combinations these rules will help you:

- All recipes in this book calling for gelatin are made with unflavored, granulated gelatin sold in 1-pound tins or in individual envelopes in boxes.
- Use either 1 tablespoon (7 grams) of the bulk gelatin or 1 envelope of the unflavored gelatin; either amount will gel 2 to 2½ cups of liquid.
- The basic fruit-flavored gel desserts which follow are to be molded in one 2- to 2½-cup bowl for serving by spoonfuls, or in 4 to 5 individual dessert dishes. Serve them plain, with toppings such as Phony Whipped Cream (*see* Index), or use a bit of fresh fruit as a garnish.
- Do *not* use the full 2 cups of the liquid if you want to make gel molds. Decrease the amount of water by ¼ cup; but always use the same amount of fruit juice and never less than ¼ cup cold water to soak the gelatin at the beginning of the recipe.
- When you want to add some cut or chopped fresh fruit, decrease liquid by ¼ cup, chill the mixture until it is the consistency of unbeaten egg whites, then fold in up to, but no more than, 1½ cups cut or chopped fruit. Turn into a 3-cup fancy mold or 6 individual dessert dishes. Be sure to add ½ Fruit Exchange (CHO 5 gm., and 20 Calories) to the individual fruit-flavored gel's food values.

- You can prepare whipped gels and the result will be double the amount of the basic recipes. To do this, prepare the basic fruit-flavored gelatin, turn it into a deep bowl, chill it until it is almost set but still lumpy; stir it occasionally during the chilling period. Beat it at high speed with an electric mixer until it is very frothy and three times its original volume. Turn it into a 6-cup dessert serving bowl, or into 8 individual dessert dishes. Chill until firm and garnish just before serving.

Pretty Apple Gel

This one is so delicious it needs nothing added to it. But if you are a yogurt or Phony Whipped Cream (see Index) fan, then you might want to add a "dollop."

4 servings (yield: 2 cups)   1 serving: ½ cup

2 teaspoons granulated gelatin
¼ cup cold water
½ cup boiling water
Artificial sweetener to substitute for 3 teaspoons sugar
1¼ cups unsweetened apple juice
1 teaspoon lemon juice
4 drops red food color (optional)
Fresh mint leaves if available

Soak gelatin in cold water. Add boiling water and artificial sweetener and stir until dissolved. Combine hot liquid with apple juice and lemon juice; mix well and stir in red food color. Chill in a covered bowl or jar until it is the consistency of unbeaten egg whites. Pour carefully into 4 individual dessert dishes. Chill until set. Garnish each with 2 leaves of fresh mint if available.

Nutritive values per serving: CHO 9 gm., PRO 1 gm., FAT 0, Calories 40, Sodium 1 mg.

Food Exchange per serving: 1 Fruit Exchange.

Low-sodium diets: This recipe is excellent.

Lemon Gelatin

4 servings (yield: almost 2 cups)   1 serving: scant ½ cup

2 teaspoons granulated gelatin
½ cup cold water
1 tablespoon grated lemon rind
1½ cups hot water
¼ cup fresh lemon juice, strained
¼ teaspoon pure lemon flavor
2 drops yellow food color (optional)
Artificial sweetener to substitute for 7 teaspoons sugar

Soak gelatin in ½ cup cold water; set aside. Add lemon rind to 1½ cups hot water, bring to a boil, and simmer for 5 minutes. Strain and measure 1¼ cups only to add to gelatin; stir to dissolve. Add remaining ingredients; stir to blend and dissolve artificial sweetener. Chill until partially set, stirring occasionally. Spoon into a 2-cup bowl or 4 individual dessert dishes. Chill until firm.

Nutritive values per serving: CHO 1 gm., PRO 1 gm., FAT 0, Calories 8, Sodium trace

Food Exchange per serving: Up to 1 cup may be considered "free."

Low-sodium diets: This recipe is excellent.

Orange Gelatin

4 servings (yield: almost 2 cups)   1 serving: scant ½ cup

2 teaspoons granulated gelatin
1 cup cold water
2 tablespoons grated fresh orange rind
1 cup strained fresh orange juice
¼ teaspoon pure orange flavor
3 drops red food color
3 drops yellow food color
Artificial sweetener to substitute for 3 teaspoons sugar

Soak gelatin in ¼ cup cold water; set aside. Add orange rind to ¾ cup water, bring to a boil, and simmer for 5 minutes. Strain and measure ½ cup only to add to gelatin; stir to dissolve. Add remaining ingredients; stir to blend and dissolve artificial sweetener. Chill until partially set, stirring occasionally. Spoon into a 2-cup serving bowl or 4 individual dessert dishes. Chill until firm.

Nutritive values per serving: CHO 7 gm., PRO 1 gm., FAT 0, Calories 31, Sodium 1 mg.

Food Exchange per serving: 1 Fruit Exchange.

Low-sodium diets: This recipe is excellent.

Pineapple Gelatin

4 servings (yield: 2 cups)   1 serving: ½ cup

2 teaspoons granulated gelatin
¼ cup cold water
½ cup boiling water
1 teaspoon lemon juice
1¼ cups unsweetened pineapple juice
Artificial sweetener to substitute for 3 teaspoons sugar

Soak gelatin in cold water. Add boiling water and lemon juice and stir to dissolve. Add pineapple juice and artificial sweetener; stir to dissolve. Chill until partially set, stirring occasionally. Spoon into a 2-

cup serving dessert bowl or 4 individual dessert dishes. Chill until set. A pretty garnish of a whole or sliced strawberry on each may be added.

Nutritive values per serving: CHO 11 gm., PRO 1 gm., FAT 0, Calories 47, Sodium 1 mg.

Food Exchange per serving: 1 Fruit Exchange.

Low-sodium diets: This recipe is excellent.

Apple Cherry Gel

5 servings (yield: 2½ cups)   1 serving: ½ cup

1 tablespoon granulated gelatin
½ cup cold water
½ cup boiling water
1 teaspoon lemon juice
1½ cups unsweetened apple juice
Artificial sweetener to substitute for 3 teaspoons sugar
4 to 5 drops red food color
10 sweet Bing cherries

Soak gelatin in cold water for a few minutes. Then add boiling water and lemon juice to dissolve gelatin. Add apple juice and artificial sweetener; stir until dissolved; add red food coloring. Chill until it is the consistency of unbeaten egg whites. Meanwhile, prepare cherries; remove and discard stems and stones, and cut cherries into eighths. Fold carefully into partially set apple gelatin and spoon carefully into dessert serving bowl or 5 dessert dishes. Chill until set. If desired, garnish each serving with 1 tablespoon of plain, low-fat yogurt or with Phony Whipped Cream (*see* Index).

Nutritive values per serving: CHO 11 gm., PRO 1 gm., FAT 0, Calories 49, Sodium 1 mg.

Food Exchange per serving: 1 Fruit Exchange.

Low-sodium diets: This recipe is excellent.

Chocolate Chiffon Mold

The kids aren't the only ones who like this yummy dessert!

6 servings (yield: 1 mold)   1 serving: ⅔ cup chocolate mold
                                          plus 2 ladyfinger halves

1 tablespoon granulated gelatin
½ cup cold water
3 medium eggs, separated
¼ cup (25 grams) dry cocoa
⅛ teaspoon salt
1 cup skim milk
1½ teaspoons pure vanilla
½ teaspoon pure chocolate extract
Artificial sweetener to substitute for ⅔ cup sugar
⅛ teaspoon cream of tartar
6 small (42 grams) ladyfingers

Soak gelatin in cold water. Beat egg yolks until light; add cocoa, salt, and milk; beat until smooth. Turn into the top of a double boiler. Cook over simmering water, stirring constantly until thick and smooth. Remove from heat. Add vanilla, chocolate extract, and artificial sweetener; mix well. Add chocolate mixture to gelatin and stir until gelatin is completely dissolved. Chill in refrigerator, stirring occasionally, until mixture sets to the consistency of unbeaten egg whites. Meanwhile, split ladyfingers. Place halves upright (flat side in) around outer sides of a 4-cup mold. When chocolate mixture is partially thickened, beat egg whites and cream of tartar until stiff. Fold into chocolate mixture; blend thoroughly. Carefully spoon into mold. Cover with clear plastic wrap. Chill for 3 to 4 hours or until set. Unmold onto a serving plate as you would any gelatin mixture. To serve, cut in six slices.

Nutritive values per serving: CHO 11 gm., PRO 7 gm., FAT 4
                                 gm., Calories 103, Sodium 100 mg.

Food Exchanges per serving: 1 Fruit Exchange plus 1 Low-Fat
                               Meat Exchange.

Low-sodium diets: Omit salt.

Heavenly Mold

4 servings (yield: 2 cups)   1 serving: ½ cup

1 tablespoon granulated gelatin
½ cup cold water
1½ cups buttermilk, made from skim milk
1 teaspoon grated lemon rind
1 teaspoon grated orange rind
2 teaspoons lemon juice
$\frac{1}{16}$ teaspoon mace
Artificial sweetener to substitute for ¼ cup sugar
1 maraschino cherry, quartered, or 4 small strawberries for garnish

Combine gelatin and cold water in a small bowl; place bowl in a
small amount of hot water to dissolve gelatin completely. Add to
buttermilk with all remaining ingredients except garnish; mix well.
Pour into four ½-cup molds. Chill for a few hours. Unmold into
small dessert dishes; garnish each with slices of a maraschino cherry
or a whole strawberry.

Nutritive values per serving: CHO 5 gm., PRO 5 gm., FAT 0,
                                 Calories 40, Sodium 120 mg.

Food Exchange per serving: ½ Milk Exchange.

Low-sodium diets: Substitute 1½ cups skim milk mixed with 1½
                   tablespoons additional lemon juice for the
                   buttermilk.

Port Parfait

4 servings (yield: 2 cups)   1 serving: ½ cup

1 tablespoon granulated gelatin
¼ cup cold water
½ cup boiling water
1 tablespoon lemon juice
¾ cup unsweetened orange juice
½ cup port wine
¼ teaspoon pure orange extract
¼ teaspoon almond extract
Artificial sweetener to substitute for 2 tablespoons sugar
1 small orange, peeled and sectioned

Soak gelatin in cold water; dissolve in boiling water. Add all
remaining ingredients except orange segments; mix well. Chill until it
is the consistency of unbeaten egg whites; stir gently and spoon into 4
parfait or wine glasses. Chill until set. Just before serving garnish
each with 3 orange segments.

Nutritive values per serving: CHO 11 gm., PRO 2 gm., FAT 1
                                  gm., Calories 82, Sodium 5 mg.
                                  (estimated).

Food Exchanges per serving: 1 Fruit Exchange plus 1 Fat Ex-
                                 change (to account for calories from
                                 the alcohol in the wine).

Low-sodium diets: This recipe is excellent.

Snow Pudding

6 servings (yield: 3 cups)   1 serving: ½ cup

1 tablespoon granulated gelatin
½ cup cold water
1 tablespoon grated lemon rind
¼ cup lemon juice
1¼ cups boiling water
Artificial sweetener to substitute for ½ cup sugar
2 medium egg whites
¼ teaspoon pure vanilla extract
¼ teaspoon pure lemon extract

Soak gelatin in cold water. Meanwhile, combine lemon rind, juice, and boiling water in a saucepan; bring to a boil, then remove from heat. Add softened gelatin and artificial sweetener; mix well to dissolve both. Chill until it is the consistency of unbeaten egg whites. Then add unbeaten egg whites, vanilla extract, and lemon extract. Beat with a rotary beater until it is very fluffy and holds its shape. Pile into 6 serving dishes. Chill until firm.

Nutritive values per serving: CHO 1 gm., PRO 2 gm., FAT 0, Calories 11, Sodium 14 mg.

Food Exchange per serving: Up to ½ cup may be considered "free"; 1 cup should be counted as ½ Lean Meat Exchange.

Low-sodium diets: This recipe is suitable.

Fresh Strawberry Fluff

6 servings (yield: 4 cups)   1 serving: ⅔ cup

¼ cup cold water
1 tablespoon granulated gelatin
1 tablespoon lemon juice
Artificial sweetener to substitute for 10 teaspoons sugar
¼ teaspoon pure orange flavor
1 pint (2 cups) fresh strawberries
3 egg whites
⅛ teaspoon salt

Measure water, gelatin, lemon juice, artificial sweetener, and orange flavor into a blender. Wash strawberries and remove hulls; set aside ½ cup berries. Cut remaining 1½ cups berries in quarters and add to mixture in blender. Cover; turn blender to high speed for about 30 seconds or until mixture is well blended. In a bowl beat egg whites and salt until stiff but not dry. Fold strawberry mixture carefully into egg whites; blend well. Slice remaining berries. Put a few slices in the bottom of each of 6 individual serving dishes, then a layer of strawberry mixture, then more strawberry slices, more mixture, and finish with a few strawberry slices on top as garnish. Chill in refrigerator until firm.

Nutritive values per serving: CHO 5 gm., PRO 3 gm., FAT 0, Calories 32, Sodium 66 mg.

Food Exchange per serving: 1 Vegetable Exchange.

Low-sodium diets: Omit salt.

Jelly Candy

21 servings (yield: 64 squares)   1 serving: 3 squares

2 tablespoons granulated gelatin
¾ cup cold water
1 cup boiling water
¼ cup orange juice
1 tablespoon lemon juice
1 teaspoon almond extract
½ teaspoon pure orange extract
Artificial sweetener to substitute for 1 cup sugar
Few drops red food coloring
1½ cups Rice Krispies

Soak gelatin in cold water. Add boiling water, fruit juices, both
extracts, artificial sweetener, and red food coloring; stir until gelatin
is dissolved. Chill until it is the consistency of unbeaten egg whites.
Fold in cereal; mix well. Turn into an 8-inch square pan. Chill for a
few hours. Cut into 1-inch squares.

Nutritive values per serving: CHO 2 gm., PRO 1 gm., FAT 0,
                                 Calories 12, Sodium 19 mg.

Food Exchange per serving: 1 serving may be considered "free";
                              2 servings (6 candies) should be
                              counted as ½ Fruit Exchange *or* 1
                              Vegetable Exchange.

Low-sodium diets: This recipe is suitable.

Cheese Cake

8 servings   1 serving: 1 piece, 4 by 2 inches

6 plain graham wafers (2½-by-2½-inches each)
1½ tablespoons margarine, melted
1 tablespoon granulated gelatin
½ cup cold water
⅓ cup boiling water
½ teaspoon grated lemon rind
½ cup lemon juice
Artificial sweetener to substitute for ¼ cup sugar
2 tablespoons water
2 cups (16 ounces) cream-style cottage cheese (4% fat)
½ teaspoon lemon extract
4 large strawberries

Prepare an 8-by-8-by-2-inch cake pan with vegetable pan coating (spray or solid); set aside. Make fine crumbs with graham crackers (½ cup), and mix thoroughly with melted margarine; set aside. Soak gelatin in cold water. Combine boiling water and lemon rind; add to gelatin; add lemon juice and artificial sweetener, stirring until completely dissolved. Chill until it is the consistency of unbeaten egg whites. Put 2 tablespoons water, cottage cheese, and lemon extract into a blender and cover; turn to high speed for 10 to 15 seconds. Add partially set gelatin mixture; turn to high speed 15 seconds or until well blended. Pour into prepared pan. Sprinkle graham cracker crumbs evenly over top. Wash strawberries, hull, and dry. Slice in halves lengthwise. Arrange on top of Cheese Cake so that, when cut into 8 servings (4 by 2 inches), each will have a strawberry garnish in center. Chill several hours until set.

Nutritive values per serving: CHO 7 gm., PRO 9 gm., FAT 5 gm., Calories 106, Sodium 192 mg.

Food Exchanges per serving: ½ Bread Exchange plus 1 Medium-Fat Meat Exchange.

Low-sodium diets: This recipe is suitable unless sodium restriction is severe. Use unsalted cottage cheese and margarine.

Refrigerator No-Cheese Cake

6 servings   1 serving: ⅙ cake

2 large (2½-by-5 inches) graham crackers
1 teaspoon margarine
1 tablespoon granulated gelatin
½ cup cold water
2 cups plain, low-fat yogurt
Artificial sweetener to substitute for 1 tablespoon sugar
½ cup iced water
1½ teaspoons grated lemon rind
1 egg white
½ cup (34 grams) instant nonfat dry milk powder
2 tablespoons lemon juice
1½ teaspoons pure vanilla
Artificial sweetener to substitute for 1 tablespoon sugar
3 maraschino cherries, halved, or 6 small strawberries for garnish

Put crackers in a plastic bag and tie top; crush with a rolling pin or jar to make fine crumbs. Melt margarine in the bottom of an 8- or 9-inch, round cake pan. Spread margarine evenly over bottom of pan. Sprinkle crumbs evenly on bottom only; press gently. Chill in refrigerator. Soak gelatin in cold water. Heat over boiling water to dissolve the gelatin. Combine yogurt and first measure of artificial sweetener; beat at moderate speed with rotary beaters, adding dissolved gelatin gradually. Chill until it is the consistency of unbeaten egg whites. Meanwhile, place iced water, lemon rind, egg white, and dry milk powder in a large bowl. Beat with rotary beaters until soft peaks form. Add lemon juice, vanilla, and second measure of sweetener. Beat at high speed until stiff. Fold into partially set yogurt; blend very well. Spoon mixture on top of crumbs in pan. Chill 4 hours or longer until set. To unmold, loosen around edge of mold with thin spatula right down to the bottom of pan. Place larger plate upside down on top of mold. Turn plate and pan over; cover top of pan for a few seconds with a hot cloth that has been run under hot water, then wrung out. Remove cloth and lift pan from mold. When ready to serve, garnish with cherries or strawberries, and cut into 6 equal slices.

Nutritive values per serving: CHO 12 gm., PRO 6 gm., FAT 2 gm., Calories 92, Sodium 114 mg.

Food Exchange per serving: 1 Milk Exchange.

Low-sodium diets: This recipe is suitable.

Applesauce Bar Cookies

See the Index for the section entitled "Sugar." Be guided by the advice of your doctor or diet counselor as to using this recipe on your individual diabetic diet

24 servings   1 serving: a 1¾-by-1¾-inch square

1¾ cups sifted cake flour
½ teaspoon baking soda
1 teaspoon cinnamon
½ teaspoon allspice
⅛ teaspoon cloves
½ teaspoon salt
¼ cup margarine
¾ cup sugar
1 medium egg
½ cup unsweetened canned applesauce
½ cup seedless raisins

Preheat oven to 375° F. (190° C.). Prepare bottom of an 11-by-7-inch pan with vegetable pan coating. Sift together flour, baking soda, spices, and salt. Cream margarine until soft and fluffy; beat in sugar gradually. Add egg and beat until light and fluffy. Add sifted dry ingredients and applesauce, alternately, stirring in just enough to blend well. Add raisins; stir until all ingredients are thoroughly mixed. Turn into the prepared pan. Bake about 30 minutes. Let cool on a baking rack for 10 minutes, then cut into 24 squares, each 1¾-by-1¾ inches.

Nutritive values per serving: CHO 15 gm., PRO 1 gm., FAT 2 gm., Calories 80, Sodium 98 mg.

Food Exchanges per serving: 1 Bread Exchange plus ½ Fat Exchange.

Low-sodium diets: Omit salt. Omit baking soda. Add 2 teaspoons low-sodium baking powder to dry ingredients when sifting together. Use unsalted margarine.

French Sponge Cookies

For best whipping volume, remove eggs from the refrigerator 30 minutes or more before using. Because each cookie contains almost ½ teaspoon sugar, it is advisable to check with a doctor or diet counselor as to using this recipe for a diabetic diet. It is almost impossible to formulate an acceptable cookie without using some sugar.

10 servings (yield: 40 cookies)　　　　　　　　1 serving: 4 cookies

½ cup sifted cake flour
¾ teaspoon baking powder
¼ teaspoon salt
3 medium eggs, separated
½ teaspoon almond extract
¼ teaspoon pure vanilla
6 tablespoons sugar

Preheat oven to 350° F. (180° C.). Sift together flour, baking powder, and salt. Beat egg yolks in a small bowl, rapidly, until very thick and lemon colored, adding almond and vanilla flavorings during the beating. With clean beaters, beat the egg whites until stiff and shiny; begin to add sugar, not more than 1 tablespoonful at a time, and beat constantly. Continue to beat rapidly until whites are very stiff and glossy. Gently and slowly fold in the beaten egg yolks. In same manner, fold in the dry ingredients until well mixed. Using a small spatula and a measuring tablespoon, measure and drop onto ungreased baking sheets 1 level tablespoon batter for each cookie, spacing them 2 inches apart. Bake 10 minutes until light golden in color. Remove from oven, and at once slide spatula under each cookie and transfer to wire cake rack to cool cookies. Let stand uncovered to dry and crisp. Store in a tightly covered container.

Nutritive values per serving
　(4 cookies):　　　　　　　　CHO 11 gm., PRO 2 gm., FAT 2
　　　　　　　　　　　　　　　gm., Calories 67, Sodium 94 mg.

Food Exchange per serving
　(4 cookies):　　　　　　　　1 Bread Exchange.

Low-sodium diets:　　　Omit salt. Use low-sodium baking powder.

Peanut Butter Cookies

12 servings (yield: 24 cookies)   1 serving: 2 cookies

1½ cups sifted all-purpose flour
1½ teaspoons baking powder
½ teaspoon salt
¼ cup margarine
½ cup (129 grams) creamy peanut butter
½ teaspoon grated, fresh orange rind
1½ teaspoons pure vanilla
1 egg, well beaten
⅓ cup orange juice
Artificial sweetener to substitute for 24 teaspoons sugar
¾ cup (115 grams) seedless raisins

Preheat oven to 400° F. (205° C.). Sift together flour, baking
powder, and salt. Cream together margarine, peanut butter, orange
rind, and vanilla. Add egg, orange juice, and artificial sweetener;
blend well. Add dry ingredients gradually; mix well after each
addition. Add raisins; mix well. Measure 1 level tablespoonful dough
for each cookie. Roll between hands to form ball. Place 2 inches
apart on an ungreased cookie sheet; flatten with fork. Bake about 15
minutes. Store cookies in a tightly covered tin. These cookies have
better flavor and texture 24 hours after baking.

Nutritive values per serving
   (2 cookies):   CHO 21 gm., PRO 5 gm., FAT 10
                                    gm., Calories 186, Sodium 242 mg.

Food Exchanges per serving
   (2 cookies):   1½ Bread Exchanges plus 2 Fat Ex-
                                    changes.

Low-sodium diets: Omit salt. Use low-sodium baking powder,
                     unsalted margarine, and unsalted peanut but-
                     ter.

Cream Puff Shells

These shells are lovely with pudding and fruit fillings but are also delightful stuffed with tuna or chicken salad.

9 servings   1 serving: 1 puff shell

¼ cup margarine
½ cup boiling water
1/16 teaspoon salt
½ cup sifted flour
2 large eggs

Preheat oven to 450° F. (230° C.). Prepare baking sheet with vegetable pan coating (spray or solid). Cut margarine into pieces; boil water and salt in a saucepan; add margarine and bring to a vigorous boil. Add flour all at once. Keeping heat low, stir rapidly to blend; then beat strenuously with a wooden spoon until the mixture forms a ball and pulls away from the sides of the pan. Remove from heat; allow to cool a few minutes. Add eggs, one at a time, beating vigorously after each addition. Drop 2 level tablespoons onto prepared sheet for each shell; place batter at least 2 inches apart. Bake for 10 minutes; reduce heat to 400° F. (205° C.) and continue baking until puffs are firm and browned, about 25 minutes. Transfer to wire rack; slit each puff with the tip of a sharp knife to allow steam to escape. Let cool before filling.

Nutritive values per serving
(unfilled shell):   CHO 5 gm., PRO 2 gm., FAT 6
                               gm., Calories 87, Sodium 91 mg.

Food Exchanges per serving
(unfilled shell):   ½ Bread Exchange plus 1 Fat Ex-
                               change *or* 1 Vegetable Exchange
                               plus 1 Fat Exchange.

Low-sodium diets: Omit salt. Substitute unsalted margarine.

Birthday Cake

Before preparing this for a diabetic we suggest you read the section entitled "Sugar" (see Index). Also, it is wise for the diabetic to discuss with the doctor or diet counselor the advisability of eating the small portion of this cake on very special occasions.

12 servings   1 serving: 1/12 cake

2 cups sifted cake flour
2½ teaspoons baking powder
½ teaspoon salt
6 tablespoons margarine, softened
1¼ teaspoons pure vanilla
¼ teaspoon almond extract
1 cup sugar
1 medium egg
¾ cup skim milk
½ cup Fresh Strawberry Spread or Apricot Spread (*see* Index)
1 cup Phony Whipped Cream (*see* Index)

Preheat oven to 350° F. (190° C.). Line two 8-inch-round layer cake pans with parchment paper or waxed paper. Sift together the sifted cake flour, baking powder, and salt. With an electric mixer at medium speed, cream together margarine, vanilla, and almond extract until fluffy. Add sugar gradually, beating constantly. Add egg; beat until mixture is very light and fluffy. Now, stirring with a wooden spoon, add dry ingredients alternately with milk (flour in fourths and milk in thirds), stirring after each addition only until batter is smooth. Turn into two prepared pans. Bake 25 to 30 minutes or until done. When cool, spread the ½ cup Fresh Strawberry or Apricot Spread between layers. Spread Phony Whipped Cream just on top, making several swirls and peaks with the tip of a spatula. Store in refrigerator until just before serving. If desired, when preparing the Phony Whipped Cream add a few drops of red or green food color to water to make it a delicate color. To cut a 1/12 slice, cut cake in quarters then cut each quarter in three equal pieces. This will give you 12 servings from the cake. See decorating instructions.

Nutritive values per serving: CHO 32 gm., PRO 3 gm., FAT 7 gm., Calories 199, Sodium 250 mg.

Food Exchanges per serving: 2 Bread Exchanges plus 1½ Fat Exchanges.

Low-sodium diets: Omit salt. Substitute low-sodium baking powder and unsalted margarine.

To Decorate Birthday Cake

If your diabetic diet is liberal enough to allow for another ½ Fat Exchange per piece of Birthday Cake, use either of these two favorite suggestions:

SEMISWEET CHOCOLATE BITS

Use 1 ounce (28 grams), approximately 60 pieces. After spreading Phony Whipped Cream on top of cake, either scatter chocolate bits on top surface of cake or arrange in a pattern.

CHOPPED NUTS

Use 2 tablespoons (16 grams) of chopped walnuts or pecans. Scatter on surface of Phony Whipped Cream or around edge of cake.

Nutritive values per serving
(decorated cake): CHO 32 gm., PRO 3 gm., FAT 8 gm., Calories 210, Sodium 251 mg.

Food Exchanges per serving
(decorated cake): 2 Bread Exchanges plus 2 Fat Exchanges.

Low-sodium diets: See directions under recipe for Birthday Cake.

Jeanette's Dutch Babies

This recipe is from our friend Jeanette L. White, R.D., Nutritionist of the American Diabetes Association, Inc., the Northern Illinois Affiliate. Serve this as a dessert or as a main dish for a brunch or luncheon meal. If used as a main course, double the portion.

4 servings (yield: 9-inch pancake)   1 serving: ¼ pancake

2 medium eggs
⅓ cup flour
⅓ cup skim milk
¼ teaspoon salt
¼ teaspoon grated lemon rind
1½ teaspoons sugar
1 tablespoon very soft margarine

Preheat oven to 400° F. (205° C.). Prepare an 8- or 9-inch-round cake pan with vegetable pan coating (spray or solid). Beat eggs until light yellow, then mix in remaining ingredients; beat until smooth. Pour into prepared pan. Bake 20 minutes, then reduce heat to 350° F. (180° C.) and continue baking for another 10 minutes. To serve, cut into 4 wedges and sprinkle with fresh lemon juice and garnish with lemon slices, or serve with Cooked Cranberry Sauce or Fluffy Lemon Sauce (*see* Index).

Nutritive values per serving: CHO 11 gm., PRO 5 gm., FAT 7 gm., Calories 116, Sodium 206 mg.

Food Exchanges per serving: 1 Fruit Exchange plus 1 Medium-Fat Meat Exchange.

Low-sodium diets: Omit salt. Use unsalted margarine.

Oh! Boy!
Strawberry Shortcake

6 servings   1 serving: 1 strawberry shortcake

3 cups fresh strawberries
6 Buttermilk Biscuits or Baking Powder Biscuits (*see* Index)
¾ cup Vanilla Crème Fraiche (*see* Index)

Hull and slice strawberries. Split each biscuit and arrange 2 halves on each plate. Spread ½ cup sliced strawberries over each 2 halves, and top each serving with 2 tablespoons Vanilla Crème Fraiche. Enjoy! If you like the strawberries sweetened, 1 hour before serving slice berries into a bowl. Sprinkle with artificial sweetener to substitute for 3 teaspoons sugar; mix well. Cover bowl and chill in refrigerator.

Nutritive values per serving: CHO 20 gm., PRO 3 gm., FAT 8 gm., Calories 160, Sodium 224 mg.

Food Exchanges per serving: 1 Bread Exchange plus ½ Fruit Exchange plus 1½ Fat Exchanges.*

Low-sodium diets: Modify biscuit recipe as directed.

* If desired you may substitute Phony Whipped Cream for the Vanilla Crème Fraiche and omit 1 Fat Exchange from the calculated value.

Baked Custard

If you want to unmold this Baked Custard, leave cups in the refrigerator 2 to 3 extra hours.

4 servings (yield: 2 cups)   1 serving: ½ cup

1½ cups skim milk
2 eggs, beaten slightly
2 tablespoons sugar (It's OK, it's in the calculated value.)
⅛ teaspoon salt
1 teaspoon pure vanilla
⅛ teaspoon grated nutmeg (optional)

Preheat oven to 325° F. (165° C.). Heat milk in the top of a double boiler over simmering water until surface begins to wrinkle. Blend together the eggs, sugar, salt, and vanilla. Add hot milk gradually, stirring to mix well. Pour into four 6-ounce individual custard cups. Sprinkle surface lightly with nutmeg. Set cups in a deep pan; pour hot water around cups to come to within ½ inch of tops of custard cups. Bake 50 to 60 minutes or until knife tip inserted in center of custard comes out clean. Remove from heat and water pan. Chill for several hours before serving.

Nutritive values per serving: CHO 10 gm., PRO 6 gm., FAT 3 gm., Calories 92, Sodium 141 mg.

Food Exchanges per serving: 1 Fruit Exchange plus 1 Lean Meat Exchange.

Low-sodium diets: Omit salt.

Bread Pudding

Use white or whole wheat bread for this old favorite. Two slices are ample for this recipe.

4 servings (yield: 3 cups)   1 serving: ¾ cup

2 slices bread
2 teaspoons margarine, softened
2 tablespoons seedless raisins
2 cups skim milk
2 eggs
¼ teaspoon salt
2 tablespoons sugar
¼ teaspoon cinnamon
1 teaspoon pure vanilla

Preheat oven to 350° F. (180° C.). Prepare a 1½-quart casserole with vegetable pan coating (spray or solid). Spread bread with margarine and cut each slice into 16 cubes. Place bread cubes in bottom of prepared casserole. Scatter raisins on top evenly. Scald (heat) milk in the top of a double boiler over simmering water; remove from heat. Beat eggs until light; beat in remaining ingredients. Pour hot milk on top, stirring to blend well; pour carefully on top of bread cubes. Place casserole in a pan of hot water (enough to come up to half of the depth of the casserole). Bake 50 minutes or until knife inserted halfway between center and outside edge comes out clean. Remove dish from water, chill pudding in refrigerator 3 hours or longer or serve warm. Serve plain or with Fluffy Lemon Sauce or Phony Whipped Cream (*see* Index).

Nutritive values per serving: CHO 23 gm., PRO 9 gm., FAT 5 gm., Calories 171, Sodium 452 mg.

Food Exchanges per serving: 1 Milk Exchange plus 1 Fruit Exchange plus 1 Fat Exchange.

Low-sodium diets: Omit salt. Substitute low-sodium bread and unsalted margarine.

Chocolate Pudding Mix

This recipe makes 2 cups of mix to be stored in a tightly covered jar on the kitchen shelf. Because cornstarch packs down tightly and cocoa packs very lightly when measured, please follow the directions for measuring exactly as given. Otherwise, you won't get the proper weights or nutritive values—or good pudding desserts!

Servings depend on use (yield: 2 cups of mix)

1 cup (68 grams) instant nonfat dry milk granules
½ cup (64 grams) lightly packed cornstarch
½ cup (43 grams) firmly packed cocoa

Sift ingredients together at least three times and mix with a fork. Pack firmly into a pint jar. Cover tightly. Store in a cool, dry place. Use for making Chocolate Pudding, Hot Chocolate Sauce, or as filling for Cream Puff Shells (*see* Index).

Nutritive values of total
   recipe: CHO 113 gm., PRO 32 gm., FAT 9 gm., Calories 590, Sodium 360 mg.

Food Exchanges per serving: Depends on use. (See following recipe for Chocolate Pudding.)

Low-sodium diets: Use low-sodium nonfat dry milk.

Chocolate Pudding from Our Mix

4 servings (yield: 2 cups)   1 serving: ½ cup

1 cup Chocolate Pudding Mix (*see* preceding recipe), firmly packed
2 cups cold water
½ teaspoon pure vanilla
Artificial sweetener to substitute for 8 teaspoons sugar

Measure dry pudding mix into a small, heavy saucepan. Add water slowly, mixing well. Stir constantly over moderate heat until bubbling boil is reached around outside edge. Remove from heat. Stir in vanilla and artificial sweetener; blend well. Pour ½ cup into each of 4 dessert dishes. Cover lightly and chill.

Nutritive values per serving: CHO 14 gm., PRO 4 gm., FAT 1 gm., Calories 73, Sodium 45 mg.

Food Exchange per serving: 1 Bread Exchange.

Low-sodium diets: Use low-sodium nonfat dry milk in Chocolate Pudding Mix.

Chocolate Milk Pudding

4 servings (yield: 2 cups)   1 serving: ½ cup

1 cup Chocolate Pudding Mix (*see* Index), firmly packed
2 cups skim milk
½ teaspoon pure vanilla
Artificial sweetener to substitute for 8 teaspoons sugar

Measure dry pudding mix into a small, heavy saucepan. Add milk slowly, mixing well. Be sure all lumps are removed. Stir constantly over medium heat until a full bubbling boil is reached. Remove from heat. Stir in vanilla and sweetener; blend well. Pour ½ cup into each of 4 small dessert dishes. Cover lightly and chill until firm. May be served with 1 tablespoon Phony Whipped Cream (*see* Index).

Nutritive values per serving: CHO 20 gm., PRO 8 gm., FAT 1 gm., Calories 118, Sodium 109 mg.

Food Exchanges per serving: 1 Milk Exchange plus ½ Bread Exchange *or* 1 Milk Exchange plus 1 Fruit Exchange.

Low-sodium diets: Use low-sodium nonfat dry milk powder in the Chocolate Pudding Mix and in this recipe.

Cranberry Tapioca Pudding

4 servings (yield: 2 cups)   1 serving: ½ cup

2 tablespoons quick-cooking tapioca
1½ cups water
2 cups fresh cranberries
½ teaspoon pure orange extract
Artificial sweetener to substitute for ½ cup sugar

Combine tapioca and water in a saucepan; let stand 5 minutes. Bring
to a boil and simmer 3 minutes, stirring frequently. Add cranberries
and cook until all berries have popped, then remove from heat. Add
orange extract and artificial sweetener, and mix well. Allow to cool
before putting in refrigerator. Chill thoroughly

Nutritive values per serving: CHO 9 gm., PRO 0, FAT 0, Calories
                                 37, Sodium 1 mg.

Food Exchange per serving: 1 Fruit Exchange.

Low-sodium diets: This recipe is excellent.

Light Pudding Mix

*This mix may be used as a base to prepare light puddings such as vanilla or
orange puddings. Be sure to measure cornstarch lightly.*

Servings depend on use (yield: 1½ cups of dry pudding mix)

1 cup (68 grams) instant nonfat dry milk granules
½ cup (64 grams) lightly packed cornstarch

Sift dry milk granules and cornstarch together three times and mix
with a fork. Pack into a pint jar; cover tightly. Store in a cool, dry
place.

Nutritive values of total
    recipe: CHO 91 gm., PRO 24 gm., FAT 0,
                             Calories 475, Sodium 358 mg.

Food Exchanges per serving: Depends on use. (See following rec-
                               ipe for Vanilla Pudding.)

Low-sodium diets: Use low-sodium nonfat dry milk.

Vanilla Pudding

If you don't use fruit, just before serving pudding put 1 teaspoon of one of the sweet spreads (see Index) on top after chilling for color and added flavor.

4 servings (yield: 2 cups)   1 serving: ½ cup

½ cup Light Pudding Mix (see preceding recipe), firmly packed
2 cups cold water
4 eggs, beaten
2 teaspoons pure vanilla
Artificial sweetener to substitute for 6 teaspoons sugar

Measure pudding mix into a small, heavy saucepan. Add water slowly, mixing well. Stir constantly over moderate heat until a bubbling boil is reached; remove from heat. Slowly pour on top of beaten eggs, stirring constantly. Return to saucepan; cook and stir over low heat 1 to 2 minutes until thick and smooth. Remove from heat; stir in vanilla and artificial sweetener until dissolved and blended. Pour ½ cup into each of 4 dessert dishes. Cover lightly and chill. For variety, place a few slices of strawberries or small pieces of orange segments or 2 tablespoons diced bananas or other fresh fruit in bottom of dessert dishes before spooning in hot, cooked pudding and chilling.*

Nutritive values per serving: CHO 8 gm., PRO 8 gm., FAT 5 gm., Calories 112, Sodium 84 mg.

Food Exchanges per serving: 1 Milk Exchange* plus 1 Fat Exchange.

Low-sodium diets: Use low-sodium nonfat dry milk in pudding mix.

* The added carbohydrate of the fruit will bring the total value of the pudding closer to the 12 grams allowed in the allotted Milk Exchange.

Rice Pudding

When you measure the rice for this recipe, weigh out 145 grams of cooked rice.

4 servings (yield: 3 cups)   1 serving: ¾ cup

2 cups skim milk
2 medium eggs, beaten
2 tablespoons sugar (It's OK, it is in the calculation.)
¼ teaspoon salt
¼ teaspoon cinnamon
1 teaspoon pure vanilla
1 cup (145 grams) cold cooked rice
2 tablespoons seedless raisins

Preheat oven to 350° F. (180° C.). Prepare a 1-quart casserole with vegetable pan coating (spray or solid). Scald (heat) milk in the top of a double boiler over simmering water. Combine eggs, sugar, salt, cinnamon, and vanilla. Pour hot milk on top slowly, stirring to mix well. Spread rice in the bottom of the casserole; scatter raisins evenly over rice; pour milk mixture carefully on top. Place casserole in pan of hot water with hot water coming almost up to the top of the casserole. Bake about 45 minutes or until knife tip inserted in center comes out clean. Remove casserole from water and chill in refrigerator. This pudding may be served warm or chilled, as you prefer. This pudding is also good topped with 1 teaspoon of one of the sweet spreads (*see* Index).

Nutritive values per serving: CHO 24 gm., PRO 8 gm., FAT 3 gm., Calories 155, Sodium 355 mg.

Food Exchanges per serving: 1 Milk Exchange plus 1 Fruit Exchange plus ½ Fat Exchange.

Low-sodium diets: Omit salt when cooking rice; omit salt in recipe.

Tapioca Nectar Fluff

5 servings (yield: 2½ cups)   1 serving: ½ cup

¼ cup quick-cooking tapioca
1 can (12 ounces) low-calorie apricot-pineapple
   nectar (no sugar added)
1 tablespoon lemon juice
¾ cup water
1 egg yolk, beaten
Artificial sweetener to substitute for ½ cup sugar
½ teaspoon pure vanilla
¼ teaspoon pure orange extract
1 egg white
3 maraschino cherries, thinly sliced

Mix tapioca, fruit nectar, lemon juice, water, and beaten egg yolk in a heavy pan; let stand 5 minutes. Bring to a full boil over medium heat; cook and stir constantly 6 to 8 minutes. Remove from heat; add sweetener and flavorings; mix well. Beat egg white to soft peaks. Gradually add tapioca, stirring quickly only until blended. Serve warm or chilled. Garnish with sliced maraschino cherries.

Nutritive values per serving: CHO 13 gm., PRO 1 gm., FAT 1
   gm., Calories 67, Sodium 11 mg.

Food Exchange per serving: 1 Bread Exchange.

Low-sodium diets: This recipe is suitable.

Hot Chocolate Sauce

This recipe is a response to the many requests from diabetics for a chocolate sauce.

6 servings (yield: 1½ cups)   1 serving: ¼ cup

½ cup Chocolate Pudding Mix (*see* Index)
1½ cups cold water
1 teaspoon pure vanilla
Artificial sweetener to substitute for 4 teaspoons sugar
½ teaspoon chocolate extract (optional)

Measure Chocolate Pudding Mix into a small, heavy saucepan. Add water gradually, mixing well. Cook and stir constantly over moderate heat until bubbling boil is reached. Remove from heat; add vanilla, artificial sweetener, and chocolate extract; mix thoroughly. Serve very warm.

Nutritive values per serving: CHO 5 gm., PRO 1 gm., FAT 0, Calories 24, Sodium 15 mg.

Food Exchange per serving: 1 Vegetable Exchange *or* ½ Fruit Exchange.

Low-sodium diets: This recipe is suitable.

Fluffy Lemon Sauce

Lovely over angel food cake, ladyfingers, or poached fruit!

7 servings (yield: 1¾ cups)   1 serving: ¼ cup

1 teaspoon granulated gelatin
2 tablespoons cold water
1 cup buttermilk (made from skim milk)
2 tablespoons lemon juice
1 teaspoon grated lemon rind
Artificial sweetener to substitute for 2 tablespoons sugar
1 medium egg white
Dash of salt

Soak gelatin in cold water, then dissolve over hot water. In a bowl combine buttermilk, lemon juice, rind, and artificial sweetener and blend well. Add the completely dissolved gelatin and mix. Chill until mixture begins to thicken. Beat egg white and salt until stiff but not dry. With a rubber spatula carefully fold egg white into buttermilk mixture. Chill.

Nutritive values per serving: CHO 2 gm., PRO 2 gm., FAT 0, Calories 17, Sodium 70 mg.

Food Exchange per serving: Up to ¼ cup may be considered "free."

Low-sodium diets: Omit salt. Substitute 1 cup skim milk mixed with 1 tablespoon additional lemon juice for the buttermilk.

Strawberry Sauce

2 servings (yield: 1⅓ cups)   1 serving: ⅔ cup

1½ cups fresh, whole strawberries
Artificial sweetener to substitute for 2 teaspoons sugar (optional)
1 tablespoon water

Wash berries; remove hulls and bad spots. (Prepared, they will weigh 225 grams.) Cut berries into bite-sized pieces. Place in a bowl, crushing bottom layer slightly with a fork. If desired, add sweetener, mixing thoroughly with water, then adding to berries, and mix well. Cover lightly. Chill until required. Serve on Baking Powder Biscuits, **Buttermilk Biscuits** (*see* Index), or ladyfingers. This sauce is also very nice with Tapioca Nectar Fluff or Rice Pudding (*see* Index).

Nutritive values per serving: CHO 9 gm., PRO 1 gm., FAT 0, Calories 40, Sodium 1 mg.

Food Exchange per serving: 1 Fruit Exchange.

Low-sodium diets: This recipe is **excellent**.

Phony Whipped Cream

24 servings (yield: 3 cups)   1 serving: 2 tablespooı

1 teaspoon granulated gelatin
1 tablespoon cold water
2½ tablespoons boiling water
½ cup iced water
½ cup instant nonfat dry milk
Artificial sweetener to substitute for 3 tablespoons sugar
½ teaspoon pure vanilla
2 tablespoons vegetable oil

Chill a small mixing bowl and beaters. Meanwhile, soften gelatin in cold water, then dissolve it over boiling water. Allow it to cool until tepid. Place iced water and nonfat dry milk in chilled bowl and beat at high speed until stiff peaks form. Continue beating, adding remaining ingredients and gelatin, until blended. Place bowl in freezer for 15 minutes, then transfer to refrigerator. Occasionally stir gently to keep mixture smooth and well blended.

Nutritive values per serving;   CHO 1 gm., PRO 1 gm., FAT 1 gm., Calories 15, Sodium 7 mg.

Food Exchange per serving: Up to 2 tablespoons may be considered "free."

Low-sodium diets: This recipe is suitable.

Vanilla Crème Fraiche

6 servings (yield: ¾ cup)   1 serving: 2 tablespoons

¼ cup whipping cream
¼ cup plain, low-fat yogurt
1 teaspoon pure vanilla

In a small chilled bowl whip cream until almost stiff. Gently fold in the yogurt and vanilla. Chill in a covered container at least two hours to allow flavors to blend. Use as topping for berries, other fruits, and desserts.

Nutritive values per serving: CHO 1 gm., PRO 0.5 gm., FAT 4 gm., Calories 41, Sodium 8 mg.

Food Exchange per serving: 1 Fat Exchange.

Low-sodium diets: This recipe is suitable.

35

Beverages

Borscht Cocktail

4 servings (yield: 2 cups)   1 serving: ½ cup

1¼ cups beet liquid (drained from canned beets)
¾ cup tomato juice
¼ teaspoon onion powder
¼ teaspoon salt
1 tablespoon lemon juice
¼ cup plain, low-fat yogurt

Mix all ingredients except yogurt. Chill 2 to 3 hours in a covered jar. Serve in cocktail glasses, topping each with 1 tablespoon yogurt.

Nutritive values per serving: CHO 7 gm., PRO 1 gm., FAT 0, Calories 34, Sodium 399 mg.

Food Exchange per serving: 1 Vegetable Exchange.

Low-sodium diets: This recipe is not suitable.

Champagne Fooler

Bubble, bubble, no toil, no trouble!

1 serving   1 serving: ¾ cup

⅓ cup chilled, unsweetened apple juice
¼ teaspoon lemon juice
Club soda, chilled

Chill a champagne glass or wine glass. Measure apple and lemon juices into a measuring cup. Add enough club soda to make a total of ¾ cup mixture; stir gently to blend. Pour into chilled champagne or wine glass. Serve immediately.

Nutritive values per serving: CHO 10 gm., PRO 0, FAT 0, Calories 40, Sodium trace.

Food Exchange per serving: 1 Fruit Exchange.

Low-sodium diets: This recipe is suitable.

Lemon Fizz

2 servings   1 serving: 1 large glass

6 ice cubes
⅓ cup lemon juice
Artificial sweetener to substitute for 6 teaspoons sugar
1 bottle (10 ounces) club soda
2 slices lemon

Crush ice cubes and divide between two 10-ounce glasses. Dissolve sweetener in lemon juice, then pour 2½ tablespoons of mixture on top of crushed ice. Pour half bottle club soda into each glass; stir briskly. Cut lemon slices halfway through to core and garnish side of each glass with a lemon slice.

Nutritive values per serving: CHO 3 gm., PRO 0, FAT 0, Calories 10, Sodium 25 mg.

Food Exchange per serving: One large glass may be considered "free."

Low-sodium diets: This recipe is suitable.

Lime Fizz

If you like Fresca, you'll love this refresher.

2 servings   1 serving: 1 large glass

6 ice cubes
¼ cup fresh or bottled, unsweetened lime juice
Artificial sweetener to substitute for 6 teaspoons sugar
1 bottle (10 ounces) club soda

Crush ice cubes and divide between two 10-ounce glasses. Dissolve sweetener in lime juice, then pour 2 tablespoons of mixture on top of crushed ice. Pour half bottle club soda on top of each; stir briskly with spoon. Serve immediately.

Nutritive values per serving: CHO 1 gm., PRO 0, FAT 0, Calories 4, Sodium 30 mg.

Food Exchange per serving: One large glass may be considered "free."

Low-sodium diets: This recipe is suitable.

Orange Fizz

2 servings   1 serving: 1 large glass

6 ice cubes
½ cup orange juice
1 teaspoon lemon juice
½ teaspoon pure orange flavor
Artificial sweetener to substitute for 2 teaspoons sugar (optional)
1 bottle (10 ounces) club soda
1 thin slice orange

Crush ice cubes and divide between two 10-ounce glasses. Mix together orange juice, lemon juice, and orange flavor; dissolve sweetener in fruit juices. Pour ¼ cup of mixed juices into each glass. Pour half bottle club soda into each glass. Stir briskly. Cut orange slice in half crosswise, then fit onto edge of glass. Serve immediately.

Nutritive values per serving: CHO 6 gm., PRO 0, FAT 0, Calories 28, Sodium 26 mg.

Food Exchange per serving: ½ Fruit Exchange.

Low-sodium diets: This recipe is suitable.

Tomato Fizz

2 servings   1 serving: ¾ cup

4 ice cubes
1 cup chilled tomato juice
2 teaspoons lemon juice
2 teaspoons Worcestershire sauce
½ teaspoon celery salt
⅔ cup club soda

Put ice cubes in two 10-ounce beverage glasses. Combine tomato juice, lemon juice, Worcestershire sauce, and celery salt; mix well. Pour on top of ice cubes. Add club soda and stir vigorously with spoon. Serve immediately.

Nutritive values per serving: CHO 6 gm., PRO 1 gm., FAT 0, Calories 24, Sodium 952 mg.

Food Exchange per serving: 1 Vegetable Exchange.

Low-sodium diets: Omit celery salt. Use unsalted tomato juice and low-sodium Worcestershire sauce.

Foamy Orange Cup

2 servings   1 serving: ¾ cup

½ cup skim milk (or buttermilk made from skim milk)
½ cup unsweetened orange juice
Artificial sweetener to equal 1 teaspoon sugar
¼ teaspoon vanilla extract
⅛ teaspoon almond extract
Dash of salt
3 ice cubes, cracked into small pieces

Place all ingredients in blender; cover. Blend on low speed until ice cubes are crushed and the drink is foamy.

Nutritive values per serving: CHO 10 gm., PRO 3 gm., FAT 0, Calories 52, Sodium 113 mg.

Food Exchanges per serving: ½ Milk Exchange plus ½ Fruit Exchange.

Low-sodium diets: Omit salt.

Pink Lady

2 servings   1 serving: ¾ cup

1 cup skim milk
3 ice cubes, cracked into small pieces
½ teaspoon imitation rum extract
1 to 2 drops red food color
Artificial sweetener to equal 1 teaspoon sugar
⅛ teaspoon vanilla extract

Chill serving glasses. Measure all ingredients into blender container; cover. Blend at low speed, then switch to high until ice cubes are crushed and mixture is foamy and well blended. Pour into glasses.

Nutritive values per serving: CHO 6 gm., PRO 4 gm., FAT 0, Calories 44, Sodium 64 mg

Food Exchange per serving: ½ Milk Exchange.

Low-sodium diets: This recipe is suitable.

Chocolate-Flavored Syrup

10 to 20 servings   1 serving: 1 to 2 tablespoons

½ cup (43 grams) dry cocoa, firmly packed
1¼ cups cold water
¼ teaspoon salt
Artificial sweetener to substitute for ½ cup sugar
2½ teaspoons pure vanilla

Mix cocoa, water, and salt in a heavy saucepan until smooth. Bring to a boil, simmer gently, stirring constantly for 3 minutes. Remove from heat; let cool 10 minutes. Add artificial sweetener and vanilla, mix well. Pour into a jar, cover, and store in refrigerator. Stir well in jar before measuring to use.

Nutritive values per serving
  (1 tablespoon):   CHO 1 gm., PRO 0, FAT 0, Calories 6, Sodium 28 mg.

Food Exchange per serving: Up to 2 tablespoons may be considered "free." If ¼ cup is used count as 1 Vegetable Exchange *or* ½ Fruit Exchange.

Low-sodium diets: Omit salt.

CHOCOLATE-FLAVORED DRINKS

These chocolate-flavored drinks are all made using the Chocolate-Flavored Syrup recipe on page 327. You may use 1 to 2 tablespoons of the Chocolate-Flavored Syrup, depending upon your own taste for chocolate.

Hot Milk Chocolate

1 serving   1 serving: 8 ounces

1 cup (8 ounces) skim milk
1 to 2 tablespoons Chocolate-Flavored Syrup (see preceding recipe)

Heat together in the top of a double boiler over simmering water, stirring frequently until very hot. Serve immediately in a warmed mug or cup.

Nutritive values per serving
(1 tablespoon syrup):   CHO 14 gm., PRO 9 gm., FAT 1 gm., Calories 94, Sodium 155 mg.

Food Exchange per serving: 1 Milk Exchange.

Low-sodium diets: Use low-sodium nonfat dry milk (reconstituted). Omit salt in Chocolate-Flavored Syrup recipe.

Double Chocolate Soda

1 serving   1 serving: 8 to 10 ounces

2 to 3 ice cubes, cracked in small pieces
2 tablespoons Chocolate-Flavored Syrup (*see* Index)
6 ounces chilled club soda

Place ice cubes in a tall beverage glass. Measure Chocolate-Flavored Syrup on top of ice. Add club soda slowly; stir vigorously with a long-handled beverage spoon to blend well. Serve at once.

Nutritive values per serving: CHO 2 gm., PRO 1 gm., FAT 1 gm., Calories 11, Sodium 86 mg.

Food Exchange per serving: One serving may be considered "free."

Low-sodium diets: Omit salt in Chocolate-Flavored Syrup recipe.

Chocolate Milk

1 serving   1 serving: 8 ounces

1 cup chilled skim milk
1 to 2 tablespoons Chocolate-Flavored Syrup (*see* Index)

Combine ingredients in a tall, cold glass and stir vigorously to mix well.

Nutritive values per serving
  (1 tablespoon syrup):   CHO 14 gm., PRO 9 gm., FAT 1 gm., Calories 94, Sodium 155 mg.

Food Exchange per serving: 1 Milk Exchange.

Low-sodium diets: Use low-sodium nonfat dry milk (reconstituted). Omit salt in Chocolate-Flavored Syrup recipe.

Mocha Milk Drink

1 serving   1 serving: 8 ounces

1 tablespoon Chocolate-Flavored Syrup (*see* Index)
1 teaspoon instant coffee powder
1 cup (8 ounces) skim milk

Measure Chocolate-Flavored Syrup into a tall glass, add instant coffee, and pour milk on top slowly, stirring vigorously to blend well. If you have a blender, measure ingredients into blender, cover, and mix at low speed for about 30 seconds.

Nutritive values per serving
  (of 8 ounces):   CHO 14 gm., PRO 9 gm., FAT 1 gm., Calories 94, Sodium 155 mg.

Food Exchange per serving: 1 Milk Exchange.

Low-sodium diets: Use low-sodium nonfat dry milk (reconstituted). Omit salt in Chocolate-Flavored Syrup recipe.

36

Little Extras

SAUCES

Barbecue Sauce

4 servings (yield: 1 cup)   1 serving: ¼ cup

½ cup finely cut onions
¼ cup finely cut sweet green peppers
½ cup water
⅓ cup catsup
3 tablespoons vinegar
2 teaspoons Worcestershire sauce
2 to 3 drops hot pepper sauce

Cook onions and green pepper in water over low heat about 8 minutes, stirring frequently. Add remaining ingredients and mix well; cook 2 more minutes.

Nutritive values per serving: CHO 9 gm., PRO 1 gm., FAT 0, Calories 36, Sodium 278 mg.

Food Exchange per serving: 1 Fruit Exchange.

Low-sodium diets: Use dietetic unsalted catsup and low-sodium Worcestershire sauce.

Caper Sauce

6 servings (yield: ¾ cup)   1 serving: 2 tablespoons

⅔ cup plain, low-fat yogurt
1 tablespoon capers, drained
1 tablespoon prepared mustard
1 tablespoon lemon juice
½ teaspoon Worcestershire sauce
3 drops liquid hot pepper sauce
¼ teaspoon salt

Combine all ingredients; turn into a half-pint jar; cover. Chill a few hours before serving. Serve as dip for chilled cooked scallops or shrimp or as a topping on seafood cocktails.

Nutritive values per serving: CHO 2 gm., PRO 1 gm., FAT 0, Calories 15, Sodium 170 mg.

Food Exchange per serving: Up to 2 tablespoons may be considered "free."

Low-sodium diets: This recipe is not suitable.

Caper Egg Sauce

4 servings (yield: 1 cup)   1 serving: ¼ cup

4 teaspoons margarine
1 tablespoon flour
½ teaspoon dry mustard
1 teaspoon salt
½ cup skim milk
½ cup fish-poaching liquid, strained
1 hard-cooked egg, finely chopped
1 tablespoon capers, drained

Melt margarine. Stir in the flour, mustard, and salt, and mix until it is smooth. Add milk and poaching liquid slowly, stirring constantly, until thick and smooth. Remove from heat; stir in egg and capers.

Nutritive values per serving: CHO 3 gm., PRO 3 gm., FAT 5 gm., Calories 70, Sodium 655 mg.

Food Exchanges per serving: 1 Fat Exchange plus 1 Vegetable Exchange.

Low-sodium diets: This recipe is not suitable.

Cooked Cranberry Sauce

This is a soft sauce or spread. If you want it firm enough to mold, increase the amount of granulated gelatin.

8 servings (yield: 4 cups)   1 serving: ½ cup

1 pound fresh or frozen cranberries
2½ cups cold water
1 teaspoon fresh grated orange rind
2 teaspoons granulated gelatin
½ teaspoon pure orange flavor
Artificial sweetener to substitute for ¾ cup sugar

Pick over and wash cranberries. Place in a deep saucepan with 2 cups water and orange rind. Bring to a boil and cook briskly until all berries have "popped." Meanwhile, soak gelatin in ½ cup cold water, remove cranberries from heat. Add gelatin, orange flavor, and artificial sweetener; stir until gelatin is dissolved and blended. Turn into jars, cover, chill, and store in refrigerator.

Nutritive values per serving: CHO 6 gm., PRO 1 gm., FAT 0, Calories 27, Sodium 1 mg.

Food Exchange per serving: 1 Vegetable Exchange *or* ½ Fruit Exchange. Up to 3 tablespoons may be considered "free" (10 calories).

Low-sodium diets: This recipe is excellent.

Creole Gumbo Sauce

Gumbo style requires the okra but if you prefer your creole sauce plain, just omit the okra.

6 servings (yield: 3 cups)   1 serving: ½ cup

2 tablespoons margarine
½ cup chopped onions
½ cup chopped sweet green pepper
½ cup thinly sliced okra, optional
1 can (16 ounces) tomatoes, with liquid
2 tablespoons tomato paste
1 cup tomato juice
2 tablespoons chopped green olives
$\frac{1}{16}$ teaspoon cayenne pepper
½ teaspoon salt
2 beef bouillon cubes
1½ teaspoons sugar

Melt margarine in a heavy saucepan; add onions, green pepper, and okra; cook gently, stirring frequently until onions are tender. Cut up tomatoes and add with tomato liquid; add all other ingredients to onion mixture; mix well. Bring to a boil; simmer gently for 8 to 10 minutes.   This sauce might be served with braised veal cutlets, broiled or baked fish, or used in making Shrimp Creole (*see* Index).*

Nutritive values per serving: CHO 9 gm., PRO 2 gm., FAT 5 gm.,
                                 Calories 83, Sodium 854 mg.
Food Exchanges per serving: 2 Vegetable Exchange plus 1 Fat
                               Exchange.
Low-sodium diets: This recipe is not suitable.

* Because veal, fish, and shrimp are particularly low in fat, count ½ cup Creole Sauce only as 2 Vegetable Exchanges and do not count the fat value.

Cucumber Sauce

7 servings (yield: 1⅔ cups)   1 serving: 2 ounces (4 tablespoons)

Puree the Cucumber Salad (*see* Index) at low speed in blender until thoroughly chopped. Chill mixture one hour before serving. This is wonderful over poached fish or over chilled canned salmon.

Nutritive values per serving: CHO 3 gm., PRO 1 gm., FAT 1 gm., Calories 22, Sodium 171 mg.

Food Exchange per serving: ½ Vegetable Exchange. Half a serving, or 1 ounce (2 tablespoons), may be considered "free."

Low-sodium diets: Omit salt in Cucumber Salad recipe.

Curry Sauce

8 servings (yield: 2 cups)   1 serving: ¼ cup

2 tablespoons margarine
1 cup thinly sliced mushrooms
¼ cup chopped onion
2 tablespoons flour
1 chicken bouillon cube
1 teaspoon salt
1½ teaspoons curry powder
1 cup skim milk
1 cup water
1 cup finely diced red apple, with skin
1½ tablespoons dried parsley or ¼ cup minced, fresh parsley

Melt margarine and add mushrooms and onions; sauté until onions are tender, stirring frequently. Stir in the flour, bouillon cube, salt, and curry powder; mix well. Add milk and water gradually, stirring until smooth. Add apple and parsley; boil gently until mixture is thick and apples are tender but not mushy. This may be served with baked or broiled chicken and hot, cooked rice.

Nutritive values per serving: CHO 7 gm., PRO 1 gm., FAT 3 gm., Calories 60, Sodium 310 mg.

Food Exchanges per serving: ½ Bread Exchange plus ½ Fat Exchange.

Low-sodium diets: Omit salt. Use unsalted margarine and low-sodium chicken bouillon cube.

Dill Sauce

This sauce is especially recommended to be served on cooked cauliflower, peas, broccoli, small boiled onions, or carrots.

8 servings (yield: 1½ cups)   1 serving: 3 tablespoons

1½ tablespoons margarine
2 tablespoons flour
1 teaspoon seasoned salt
⅛ teaspoon white pepper
1 teaspoon instant chicken bouillon or 1 chicken bouillon cube
½ cup hot water
1 cup plain, low-fat yogurt
1 tablespoon minced, fresh dill weed or 1 teaspoon dried dill weed

Melt margarine; stir in flour, salt, and pepper, and blend until smooth. Add bouillon, then water, gradually stirring to blend. Cook over low heat, stirring constantly until thick and smooth. Remove from heat. Stir in yogurt and dill weed; blend well. Stir over low heat but do not allow to boil.

Nutritive values per serving: CHO 3 gm., PRO 1 gm., FAT 3 gm., Calories 40, Sodium 367 mg.

Food Exchange per serving: 1 Fat Exchange.

Low-sodium diets: Omit salt. Use unsalted margarine and a low-sodium chicken bouillon cube.

Hotcha Beef Sauce

4 servings (yield: 1 cup)   1 serving: ¼ cup

6 tablespoons catsup
⅓ cup vinegar
1 tablespoon prepared mustard
1 tablespoon Worcestershire sauce
½ teaspoon garlic powder
½ teaspoon crushed oregano
½ teaspoon chili powder
¼ teaspoon salt
½ cup beef consommé
¼ cup water

Combine all ingredients in a small saucepan; mix well. Bring to a boil; simmer gently for about 3 minutes to blend flavors. Delicious on minute steaks, cubed cooked beef, or sliced pot roast.

Nutritive values per serving: CHO 7 gm., PRO 1 gm., FAT 0, Calories 34, Sodium 570 mg.

Food Exchange per serving: 1 Fruit Exchange.

Low-sodium diets: Omit salt. Use unsalted catsup and low-sodium Worcestershire sauce and low-sodium beef consommé.

Real Italian Sauce

7 servings (yield: 3½ cups)   1 serving: ½ cup

1 can (12 ounces) tomato paste
2 cups water
1 can (12 ounces) V-8 Juice
1 tablespoon minced onion
1 tablespoon wine vinegar
1 teaspoon minced garlic
½ teaspoon oregano
½ teaspoon basil
Pinch of crushed red pepper

Combine all ingredients in a medium pot. Simmer gently for 25 minutes, stirring occasionally. This sauce keeps well in refrigerator or may be frozen in 1-cup containers and used as needed.

Nutritive values per serving: CHO 11 gm., PRO 2 gm., FAT 0, Calories 49, Sodium 488 mg.

Food Exchanges per serving: ½ Fruit Exchange plus 1 Vegetable Exchange, *or* 2 Vegetable Exchanges.

Low-sodium diets: Use unsalted tomato paste and replace V-8 Juice with unsalted tomato juice.

Mock Hollandaise Sauce

This is very similar to a light Hollandaise sauce. It is excellent on a variety of cooked vegetables and especially fine for making deviled eggs.

8 servings (yield: ¾ cup)   1 serving: 1½ tablespoons

1 egg yolk
¾ cup plain, low-fat yogurt
2 tablespoons lemon juice
¼ teaspoon salt
⅛ teaspoon dry mustard

Beat egg yolk slightly in a heavy saucepan with ¼ cup yogurt, lemon juice, salt, and mustard. Cook over low heat, stirring constantly until thick and smooth. Remove from heat. Slowly stir in remaining ½ cup yogurt; blend well. Serve warm over vegetables or store in a covered jar in refrigerator.

Nutritive values per serving:
  1 serving— CHO 1.5 gm., PRO 1 gm., FAT 1 gm., Calories 18, Sodium 78 mg.
  ¼ cup— CHO 4 gm., PRO 3 gm., FAT 2 gm., Calories 48, Sodium 209 mg.

Food Exchanges per serving:
  1 serving— Up to 1½ tablespoons may be considered "free."
  ¼ cup— ½ Milk Exchange plus ½ Fat Exchange.

Low-sodium diets: Omit salt.

Mustard Sauce

8 servings (yield: ½ cup)   1 serving: 1 tablespoon

2 egg yolks
½ teaspoon dry mustard
3 tablespoons white vinegar
3 tablespoons skim milk
1 tablespoon prepared mustard
1 tablespoon lemon juice
Artificial sweetener to substitute for 1 teaspoon of sugar

Beat egg yolks with dry mustard in the top of a double boiler until blended. Add vinegar gradually, beating after each addition. Cook over simmering water, stirring constantly until thick and smooth. Add milk gradually, beating in with a fork or wire whip. Cook 5 more minutes over simmering water. Remove from heat. Let cool 10 minutes. Add remaining ingredients, blend well. This is delicious served with ham, pork, or Canadian-style bacon.

Nutritive values per serving: CHO 1 gm., PRO 1 gm., FAT 1 gm., Calories 18, Sodium 28 mg.

Food Exchange per serving: Up to 1 tablespoon may be considered "free." If you use 3 tablespoons count it as 1 Fat Exchange.

Low-sodium diets: This recipe is suitable, but should be used with fresh pork, not ham or Canadian-style bacon.

Sweet and Sour Sauce

This may be served with cooked shrimp, chicken, ham or pork.

8 servings (yield: 2 cups)   1 serving: ¼ cup

1½ tablespoons cornstarch
½ teaspoon ground ginger *or* 1 teaspoon
   grated fresh ginger
¼ teaspoon salt
1 can (8½ ounces) dietetic pineapple tidbits
   canned in pineapple juice (no sugar added)
¼ cup cider vinegar
1 tablespoon soy sauce
1¼ cups chicken broth
Artificial sweetener to substitute for ¼ cup sugar

Mix cornstarch, ginger, and salt in a small, heavy saucepan. Drain pineapple tidbits saving liquid; set pineapple aside. Combine drained pineapple liquid, vinegar, soy sauce, and chicken broth; add gradually to cornstarch mixture, stirring until smooth. Bring to a boil and cook over medium heat, stirring constantly until thick and smooth. Add pineapple; simmer gently 4 to 5 minutes.

Nutritive values per serving: CHO 6 gm., PRO 1 gm., FAT 0, Calories 25, Sodium 345 mg.

Food Exchange per serving: ½ Fruit Exchange *or* 1 Vegetable Exchange.

Low-sodium diets: This recipe is not suitable.

FATS

Low-Fat Whipped Butter

This recipe is for readers who live in areas where a whipped butter spread is not available. Whipped butter has a lower fat and calorie count than solid butter. This recipe goes back in Kay's family at least four generations. Her first experience with it was in the '30s during the Depression, then again during World War II when butter was rationed. It is recommended only as a low-fat, low-calorie spread and is never to be used in cooking.

64 tablespoons (yield: 4 cups)   1 serving: 1 teaspoon

1 teaspoon granulated gelatin
2 tablespoons water
1 pound butter, softened
½ teaspoon salt
2 cups skim milk
Few drops yellow food color (optional)
½ teaspoon imitation butter flavor (optional)

Soak gelatin in cold water. Cut butter in very small pieces and place in a deep, warmed, dry bowl. When butter is very soft, beat with rotary egg beater or electric beater, gradually beating in gelatin and salt. Add milk slowly, beating constantly. It may take 10 minutes to beat in all the milk, but keep on beating. Add a few drops of yellow food color and imitation butter flavor toward end of beating. Beat until completely blended. Pack into containers that can be covered tightly. Store in refrigerator to harden and keep firm. Use only for spreading on bread, toast, crackers, muffins.

Nutritive values per serving: CHO 0, PRO 0, FAT 2 gm., Calories 18, Sodium 90 mg.

Food Exchange per serving
    (of 1 teaspoon):   Less than ½ Fat Exchange.

Low-sodium diets: Omit salt. Use unsalted butter. Store in coldest part of refrigerator (not freezer).

Whipped Herb Butter

1 cup Low-Fat Whipped Butter
¾ teaspoon powdered mixed herb seasonings

Mix thoroughly, cover, and refrigerate until firm. Use on cooked vegetables. For food values see values for Low-Fat Whipped Butter recipe.

Whipped Chive Butter

1 cup Low-Fat Whipped Butter
1 tablespoon finely chopped chives

Mix thoroughly, cover, and refrigerate until firm. Use on baked potatoes. For food values see values for Low Fat Whipped Butter recipe.

SWEET SPREADS

Apricot Spread

10 servings (yield: 1¼ cups)   1 serving: 2 tablespoons

2 cups prepared, fresh apricots
¾ cup water
1 teaspoon lemon juice
1½ teaspoons granulated gelatin
½ teaspoon pure almond extract
Artificial sweetener to substitute for 3 tablespoons sugar

Wash ripe apricots, cut in halves, and discard stones and dark spots. Cut halves in small, bite-sized pieces. Measure 2 cups (250 grams). Put in a heavy saucepan with ½ cup water and lemon juice. Bring to a boil; lower heat and simmer gently for 8 to 10 minutes, stirring frequently with a wooden (not metal) spoon. Meanwhile, soak gelatin in ¼ cup cold water. When apricots are cooked, remove from heat. Add gelatin, almond extract, and artificial sweetener; mix thoroughly. Pack into 2 or 3 small hot jars; cover lightly and allow to cool. Cover tightly and store in refrigerator.

Nutritive values per serving: CHO 3 gm., PRO 0.5 gm., FAT 0, Calories 14, Sodium trace.

Food Exchange per serving: Up to 2 tablespoons may be considered "free."

Low-sodium diets: This recipe is excellent.

Apple Jelly Spread

When Kay developed this recipe she said it reminded her of her grand-mother's Dolga crab apple jelly!

32 servings (yield: 2 cups)   1 serving: 1 tablespoon

2 cups unsweetened apple juice
1 teaspoon lemon juice
6 large or 8 small whole cloves
2 teaspoons granulated gelatin
½ cup water
Artificial sweetener to substitute for ¾ cup sugar
Few drops red food color (optional)

Combine apple and lemon juices and whole cloves in a heavy saucepan. Bring to a boil; simmer gently 10 minutes. Meanwhile, soak gelatin in cold water. Remove apple juice from heat; discard cloves; add gelatin and artificial sweetener and mix well to dissolve. Add about three drops red food color; mix well. Pour carefully into two hot, clean half-pint jars. Cover lightly until cooled. Then cover tightly and store in refrigerator. Spread on bread, toast, muffins, or crackers.

Nutritive values per serving: CHO 2 gm., PRO 0, FAT 0, Calories 8, Sodium trace.

Food Exchange per serving: Up to 2 tablespoons may be considered "free."

Low-sodium diets: This recipe is excellent.

Blueberry Spread

24 servings (yield: 1½ cups)   1 serving: 1 tablespoon

2 cups blueberries
¾ cup water
2 teaspoons lemon juice
1½ teaspoons granulated gelatin
Artificial sweetener to substitute for 3 tablespoons sugar

Combine blueberries, ½ cup water, and lemon juice in a heavy saucepan. Bring to a boil; simmer gently for about 8 minutes, stirring frequently. Meanwhile, soak gelatin in ¼ cup cold water. Remove blueberries from heat; add gelatin and artificial sweetener and mix well to dissolve. Turn into small, hot jars; cover lightly and allow to cool. Cover tightly and store in refrigerator. Use as a spread on bread, toast, muffins, crackers.

Nutritive values per serving: CHO 2 gm., PRO 0, FAT 0, Calories 8, Sodium trace.

Food Exchange per serving: Up to 2 tablespoons may be considered "free."

Low-sodium diets: This recipe is excellent.

Concord Grape Jelly Spread

This bread or toast spread has a real grapey flavor. You may use red or white grape juice in place of the purple if you like.

24 servings (yield: 1½ cups)   1 serving: 1 tablespoon

1½ cups pure, Concord grape juice
1 teaspoon lemon juice
2 teaspoons granulated gelatin
½ cup cold water
Artificial sweetener to substitute for ¼ cup sugar

Combine grape juice and lemon juice in a heavy saucepan. Bring to a boil; simmer 3 to 4 minutes. Meanwhile, soak gelatin in cold water. Remove grape juice from heat. Add gelatin and artificial sweetener;

mix well to dissolve. Pour into two half-pint jars, cover lightly and cool. Cover tightly and store in refrigerator. Use as a spread on bread, toast, muffins, or crackers.

Nutritive values per serving: CHO 3 gm., PRO 0, FAT 0, Calories 11, Sodium trace.

Food Exchange per serving. 1 tablespoon may be considered "free."

Low-sodium diets: This recipe is excellent.

Fresh Peach Spread

This is one of Kay's favorite toast spreads.

24 servings (yield: 1½ cups)   1 serving: 1 tablespoon

2 cups prepared fresh peaches
1 teaspoon lemon juice
¾ cup cold water
1½ teaspoons granulated gelatin
Artificial sweetener to substitute for 3 tablespoons of sugar
⅛ teaspoon pure orange extract

Select fresh, just-ripe peaches (about 1 pound). Pare peaches and remove pits. Cut peaches in small, bite-sized pieces. Measure 2 cups (370 grams). Place in a heavy saucepan with lemon juice and add ½ cup cold water. Bring to a boil; simmer gently for about 8 minutes, stirring frequently. Meanwhile, soak gelatin in ¼ cup cold water. Remove cooked peaches from heat. Add gelatin, artificial sweetener, and orange extract; mix well to blend flavors and dissolve gelatin. Turn into two or three small, hot jars; cover lightly and allow to cool. Cover tightly and store in refrigerator. Use as spread on bread, toast, muffins, crackers.

Nutritive values per serving: CHO 1 gm., PRO 0, FAT 0, Calories 7, Sodium trace.

Food Exchange per serving: Up to 2 tablespoons may be considered "free."

Low-sodium diets: This recipe is excellent.

Red Plum Spread

20 servings (yield: 1¼ cups)   1 serving: 1 tablespoon

1¼ cups prepared fresh red plums
¾ cup water
1 teaspoon lemon juice
1¼ teaspoons granulated gelatin
Artificial sweetener to substitute for 4 tablespoons sugar

Wash plums; discard stems, stones, and bad spots; cut plums in small, bite-sized pieces. Measure 1¼ cups (225 grams). Combine plums with ½ cup water and lemon juice in a heavy saucepan. Bring to a boil, then simmer gently about 8 minutes, stirring frequently. Meanwhile, soak gelatin in ¼ cup cold water. Remove cooked plums from heat; stir in gelatin and artificial sweetener and mix well. Turn into clean, small jars; cover lightly until cool. Then cover tightly and store in the refrigerator. Use as a tasty spread on bread, toast, muffins, and crackers.

Nutritive values per serving: CHO 2 gm., PRO 0, FAT 0, Calories 8, Sodium trace.

Food Exchange per serving: Up to 2 tablespoons may be considered "free."

Low-sodium diets: This recipe is excellent.

Fresh Strawberry Spread

18 servings (yield: 2¼ cups)   1 serving: 2 tablespoons

2 pints fresh strawberries
2 tablespoons cold water
1½ tablespoons lemon juice
2 teaspoons granulated gelatin
¼ cup cold water
Artificial sweetener to substitute for 12 teaspoons sugar

Wash and clean berries; discard hulls. Measure 3 cups (450 grams). Cut berries in small, bite-sized pieces and place in a heavy pan with

2 tablespoons cold water and lemon juice. Partially crush berries. Bring to a boil. Stir and cook rapidly about 5 minutes until berries are just cooked. Meanwhile, soak gelatin in ¼ cup cold water. Remove berries from heat. Add gelatin and artificial sweetener and stir to dissolve and blend. Remove scum from surface and discard. Turn into hot, small jars; cover lightly and cool. Then cover tightly and store in refrigerator. Use as spread on bread, toast, muffins, rolls.

Nutritive values per serving: CHO 2 gm., PRO 0, FAT 0, Calories 10, Sodium trace.

Food Exchange per serving: Up to 2 tablespoons may be considered "free."

Low-sodium diets: This recipe is excellent.

RELISHES

Raw Apple Relish

7 servings (yield: 1¼ cups)   1 serving: 3 tablespoons

1 medium red skin apple, cored and finely chopped
1 tablespoon lemon juice
3 tablespoons finely diced onion
2 tablespoons chopped sweet gherkins
2 tablespoons chopped ripe olives
¼ cup Low-Calorie French dressing

Combine all ingredients well. Pack into a pint container. Cover and chill for a few hours before serving.

Nutritive values per serving: CHO 5 gm., PRO 0, FAT 2 gm., Calories 33, Sodium 20 mg.

Food Exchange per serving: 1 Vegetable Exchange. Up to 1½ tablespoons may be considered "free."

Low-sodium diets: This recipe is suitable.

Pickled Beets

4 servings   1 serving: 3 small beets

1 can (8¼ ounces) whole, very small beets
¾ cup cider vinegar
1 teaspoon mixed pickling spices
1 stick cinnamon, 2 inches long
Artificial sweetener to substitute for 3 teaspoons sugar

Drain beets, saving liquid. Combine liquid and vinegar in a 1-quart pot. Add pickling spices (in a cheesecloth bag or small tea ball) and cinnamon. Bring to a boil; simmer 5 minutes. Discard spices. Pack beets into a pint jar. Dissolve sweetener in hot liquid; pour on top of beets. Cover and store in refrigerator a few days before serving.

Nutritive values per serving: CHO 7 gm., PRO 0, FAT 0, Calories 24, Sodium 95 mg.

Food Exchange per serving: 1 Vegetable Exchange. One small beet served as a garnish on a salad or cold meat plate may be considered "free."

Low-sodium diets: This recipe is not suitable because beets are quite high in sodium.

Sweet Pickled Cherries

A delightful treat for everyone, and so easy to make! Serve with a salad, as a tasty, unusual garnish, or as finger food on relish trays.

8 or more servings (yield: 1 quart,   1 serving: 7 cherries
            50 to 60 cherries)

3 cups (1 pound) sweet Bing cherries, with stems
1 cup cold water
1 cup white vinegar
1 teaspoon brown sugar
1 tablespoon salt

Pick over cherries to select firm, ripe ones. Leave on as many stems as possible. Carefully wash and drain cherries. Pack easily into a 1-

quart jar, shaking but not pressing down. Save the remaining few cherries for another use. Combine remaining ingredients until salt dissolves, then pour on top of cherries. Seal jar tightly and turn upside down. Leave for 2 hours in a cool place. Turn upright. Store in refrigerator. Do not use for at least 24 hours.

Nutritive values per serving: CHO 10 gm., PRO 0, FAT 0, Calories 37, Sodium 840 mg.

Food Exchanges per serving:
   7 cherries—1 Fruit Exchange.
   3 to 4 cherries—½ Fruit Exchange.
   1 to 2 cherries may be considered "free."

Low-sodium diets: This recipe is not suitable.

Cranberry and Orange Relish

Serve with hot or cold sliced, baked poultry or ham. To freeze this relish, omit artificial sweetener and add it at time of serving.

8 servings (yield: 1½ cups)   1 serving: 3 tablespoons

2 cups (½ pound) fresh or frozen cranberries
1 medium (190 grams) orange
Artificial sweetener to substitute for 4 tablespoons sugar

Wash and pick over cranberries; discard overripe berries. Wash orange, cut in small chunks, discard seeds and center core. Put both fruits through a food grinder using coarse blade. Add artificial sweetener; mix well. Chill in a covered container.

Nutritive values per serving: CHO 4 gm., PRO 0, FAT 0, Calories 16, Sodium trace.

Food Exchange per serving: Up to 3 tablespoons may be considered "free."

Low-sodium diets: This recipe is excellent.

Pickled Cucumber Strips

These pickles are suitable for refrigerator storage only up to one week.

8 servings (yield: 1 pint jar)   1 serving: 3 strips

3 small (about ½ pound) pickling cucumbers, 3 to 4 inches long
1 cup cider vinegar
½ cup water
1 teaspoon mixed pickling spices
½ teaspoon salt
½ teaspoon celery seed
1 stick cinnamon, 3 to 4 inches long
Artificial sweetener to substitute for 12 teaspoons sugar

Scrub cucumbers; remove and discard ends; cut cucumbers length-wise in eight strips each; set aside. Combine vinegar, water, spices, salt, celery seed, and cinnamon. Bring to a boil, turn heat low, and let simmer for 5 minutes. Add cucumber strips; return to a boil and simmer for 3 minutes. Add artificial sweetener and mix well. Pack strips upright in a hot, pint jar. Strain vinegar and pour on top of cucumber strips. Cover jar, cool, and store in refrigerator. Do not use for 24 hours. Use within week.

Nutritive values per serving.   CHO 3 gm., PRO 0, FAT 0, Calories 9, Sodium 135 mg.

Food Exchange per serving: Up to 3 strips may be considered "free."

Low-sodium diets: This recipe is not suitable.

Raisins Indienne

This is a very special treat. Kay reminds the diabetic that one serving (1 tablespoon), although small, should be eaten only occasionally. Nondiabetics will want more.

24 servings (yield: 1½ cups)   1 serving: 1 tablespoon

1 cup seedless raisins
½ cup finely cut sweet green pepper
½ cup finely cut celery
½ cup finely cut green onions
1½ tablespoons margarine
¼ cup boiling water
2 tablespoons chopped Major Grey's Chutney
¼ cup slivered, blanched almonds
3 tablespoons diced pimiento
1½ tablespoons vinegar
1½ tablespoons brown sugar

Combine first six ingredients in a heavy frying pan. Bring to a boil, turn heat low, cover, and simmer gently until crisp-tender. Add all remaining ingredients. Stir over moderate heat to blend and heat together. Serve with roast duckling, chicken, lamb, or pork, or on top of hot cooked rice (plain or curried). One tablespoon over cottage cheese adds a wonderful flavor and color contrast.

Nutritive values per serving: CHO 7 gm., PRO 0.5 gm., FAT 1 gm., Calories 40, Sodium 17 mg.

Food Exchange per serving: 1 Fruit Exchange *or* ½ Bread Exchange.

Low-sodium diets: This recipe is suitable.

Tomato Relish

12 servings (yield: 1½ cups)   1 serving: 2 tablespoons

1 can (16 ounces) tomatoes, with liquid
¼ cup finely chopped onion
1 teaspoon salt
¼ cup finely cut celery
¼ cup finely cut sweet green pepper
1 teaspoon celery seed
1 tablespoon white vinegar
Dash of cayenne
Artificial sweetener to substitute for 1 teaspoon sugar

Turn tomatoes and liquid into a small bowl; cut tomatoes into very small pieces. Add all remaining ingredients and mix well. Turn into a pint jar; cover tightly. Store in refrigerator several hours before using. Serve as relish with hot or cold meats or as a sauce on seafood cocktails. Use within a week or 10 days.

Nutritive values per serving: CHO 2 gm., PRO 1 gm., FAT 0, Calories 11, Sodium 232 mg.

Food Exchange per serving: Up to 2 tablespoons may be considered "free."

Low-sodium diets: Omit salt. Use unsalted canned tomatoes.

Dilly Vegetable Pickles

16 servings (yield: 1 pint)   1 serving: 2 tablespoons

¾ cup white vinegar
¾ cup cold water
1 teaspoon salt
1½ teaspoons dill seeds
1 cup small cauliflowerets
1 small (3 ounces) pickling cucumber
4 to 5 small, white pickling onions, peeled
Artificial sweetener to substitute for 6 teaspoons sugar

Combine vinegar, cold water, salt, and dill seeds and bring to a boil; simmer for 5 minutes. Prepare vegetables: slice cucumber crosswise and measure ¾ cup; slice onions crosswise in thin slices and separate into rings. Add cauliflowerets, cucumbers, and onions to hot vinegar; bring to a boil and cook gently for 1 minute. Remove from heat. Add artificial sweetener and stir until dissolved. Spoon vegetables carefully into a hot, clean pint jar. Pour vinegar mixture on top. Cover and cool. Seal jar and store in refrigerator. Do not use for 24 hours. Use within a week—no longer

Nutritive values per serving: CHO 1 gm., PRO 0, FAT 0, Calories 5 Sodium 134 mg.

Food Exchange per serving: Up to 2 tablespoons may be considered "free."

Low-sodium diets: This recipe is not suitable.

Sources of Information

About Diabetes

American Association of Diabetes Educators
233 East Erie St.—Suite 712
Chicago, Illinois 60611
    Their publication *The Diabetes Educator* is for diet counselors.

American Diabetes Association, Inc.
600 Fifth Avenue
New York, New York 10020
    Ask for the name of your local or state affiliate. Members receive *"Diabetes Forecast."* Request their new pamphlet *"What You Need To Know About Diabetes,"* and a list of available literature. Diet counselors may subscribe to *"Diabetes Care."*

American Diabetes Association, Northern Illinois Affiliate, Inc.
620 North Michigan Avenue
Chicago, Illinois 60611
    "Expanded Guide for Meal Planning" and *"Diet Counselors Supplement"* for additional information on food exchanges and current information on fast foods.

A Guide for Professionals: The Effective Application of "Exchange Lists for Meal Planning," American Diabetes Association, Inc. and The American Dietetic Association, 1977.
    This is the counselors' guide for calculating diets.

Biermann, June and Toohey, Barbara. *The Diabetes Question and Answer Book* (Sherbourne Press, Inc.), 1974.

Biermann, June and Toohey, Barbara. *The Diabetic's Sports and Exercise Book* (Philadelphia: J. B. Lippincott Company), 1977.

Brothers, Milton J., M. D. *Diabetes, The New Approach* (New York: Grosset & Dunlap), 1976.

Canadian Diabetic Association
1491 Yonge Street
Toronto, Ontario M4T-125
Canada

Juvenile Diabetes Foundation
23 East 26th Street
New York, New York 10010
  Ask for your local affiliate's name and address.

Nutrition & the M. D. (periodical), Vol. III, No. 2 (December 1976).
  This issue is a review of sugar and sugar substitutes.

Seventh Day Adventist Dietetic Association
P. O. Box 75
Loma Linda, California 92354
  For information about vegetarianism and the diabetic diet for the vegetarian.

Traisman, Howard S., M. D. *Management of Juvenile Diabetes Mellitus,* 3rd ed. (St. Louis: C. V. Mosby Co.), 1979.

White, Philip L. and Selvey, Nancy, R. D., eds. *Let's Talk About Food* (Department of Foods and Nutrition, American Medical Association), 1974.

Food and Food Preparation

Bloch, Barbara. *The Meat Board Meat Book,* (National Livestock and Meat Board, 444 North Michigan Avenue, Chicago, Illinois 60611), 1977.

Bowen, Angela. *The Diabetic Gourmet* (New York: Barnes & Noble), 1973.

Buying Guide for Fresh Fruits, Vegetables, Herbs and Nuts, 5th ed. (Educational Department, Blue Goose, Inc., P.O. Box 46, Fullerton, California 92632).

Comidas Hispana en Dietas Diabetica. (Visiting Nurse Association of Milwaukee, 1540 North Jefferson Street, Milwaukee, Wisconsin 53202), 1975.

Handbook of Food Preparation, 7th ed. (American Home Economics Association, 2010 Massachusetts Avenue, N.W., Washington, D.C. 20036), 1975.

How to Eye and Buy Seafood and Seafood Slimmers. (National Marketing Services Office, National Marine Fisheries Service, 100 East Ohio Street, Chicago, Illinois 60607), 1971.

Nutrient Data

Church, Charles Frederick and Church, Helen Nichols. *Food Values of Portions Commonly Used,* 12th ed. (Philadelphia: J.B. Lippincott Company), 1975.

Composition of Foods, Dairy—Egg Products, Agriculture Handbook 18-1, U.S. Dept. of Agriculture. (Washington, D.C.: Superintendent of Documents, U.S. Printing Office), 1976.

Kraus, Barbara. *The Dictionary of Sodium, Fats, and Cholesterol.* (New York: Grosset & Dunlap, New York), 1974.

Nutritive Value of American Foods in Common Units, Agriculture Handbook, 456, U.S. Dept. of Agriculture. (Washington, D.C.: Superintendent of Documents, U.S. Printing Office), 1975.

Nutritive Value of Foods, Home and Garden Bulletin 72, U.S. Dept. of Agriculture. (Washington, D.C.: Superintendent of Documents, U.S. Printing Office), 1977.

Index